CH00706512

# WHAT EVERYWOMA. ABOUT HER BREASTS

DR PATRICIA GILBERT is a Senior Clinical Medical Officer and a Medical Practitioner in Community Child Health. She was trained at St George's Hospital Medical School, London, and has both hospital and general practice experience. She is also the author of *Common Childhood Illnesses* (Sheldon Press), *Your Pregnancy Diary* (Futura), *The Baby Sitters Handbook* (Whittet Books) and co-author of *The Complete Book of Babycare* (Octopus, Marks and Spencer), and is a regular contributor to *Nursery World*. She is married, with two children.

# HEALTHCARE FOR WOMEN SERIES

**Coping with Stress**
*Georgia Witkin-Lanoil*

**Eating Well for a Healthy Pregnancy**
*Dr Barbara Pickard*

**Everything You Need to Know about the Pill**
*Wendy Cooper and Dr Tom Smith*

**How to Get Pregnant & How Not To**
*P. Bello, Dr C. Dolto and Dr A. Schiffmann*

**Lifting the Curse: How to relieve painful periods**
*Beryl Kingston*

**Menopause: A practical, self-help guide for women**
*Raewyn Mackenzie*

**Successful Breastfeeding**
*Joan Neilson*

**Taking Care of Your Skin**
*Dr Vernon Coleman*

**Thrush: How it's caused and what to do about it**
*Caroline Clayton*

**What Everywoman Should Know about Her Breasts**
*Dr Patricia Gilbert*

**Women and Depression: A practical self-help guide**
*Deidre Sanders*

**Women and Tranquillisers**
*Celia Haddon*

**Women's Problems: An A to Z**
*Dr Vernon Coleman*

**You and Your Caesarean Birth**
*Trisha Duffett-Smith*

**You and Your Premature Baby**
*Barbara Glover and Christine Hodson*

HEALTHCARE FOR WOMEN

# WHAT EVERYWOMAN SHOULD KNOW ABOUT HER BREASTS

*Dr Patricia Gilbert*

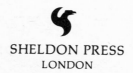

SHELDON PRESS

LONDON

First published in Great Britain in 1986 by
Sheldon Press, SPCK, Marylebone Road, London NW1 4DU

Thanks are due to Churchill Livingstone for permission to
reproduce an adapted illustration of a section of the breast from
*Textbook for Midwives* by Margaret Myles (10th Ed. 1985).

British Library Cataloguing in Publication Data

Gilbert, Patricia
    What everywoman should know about her breasts.
    ——(Healthcare for women)
    1. Breast
    I. Title    II. Series
    612'.664    QM495
ISBN 0-85969-495-X
ISBN 0-85969-496-8 Pbk

Typeset by Photobooks (Bristol) Ltd
Printed in Great Britain by
Richard Clay (The Chaucer Press) Ltd,
Bungay, Suffolk

*To Diane*
*whose valued acquaintance was made over the*
*typing of this book*

# Contents

# Introduction

Medical conditions affecting the breasts are amongst the commonest seen in doctor's surgeries. Not only lumps in the breast send women hurrying to their doctors. Infections and trauma of all kinds can also affect these organs of femininity. (But remember that men can also have breast problems. Cancer can affect the male breast—rare but possible; see Appendix.)

This book is designed to help women of all ages look after their breasts. Advice is given on a number of subjects; from what bra to choose (if any) at puberty and the care of the breasts during pregnancy, as well as the more obvious medical conditions which can affect the breasts. Part 1 covers the conditions usually seen in the 'young breast', from approximately 0 to 20 years. Part 2 covers the 'active breast', approximately between 20 and 40 years of age, when the breast is much concerned, albeit in an indirect way, in the reproductive process. Part 3 covers the 'mature breast', from 40 years of age onwards. This section includes such conditions as cysts and cancer of the breast. While the conditions described under the various headings are by no means exclusive to the age range under discussion, they will be found to occur more frequently at these times of life. For example, cancer of the breast *can* affect any woman from puberty upwards, but by far the highest incidence of this condition is in the woman of over 40. 'Self-examination' of the breasts for lumps is discussed in Chapter 4 in order that women will, as routine, examine their breasts at regular intervals, so that the tiniest lump can be found and treated as early as possible.

Breasts form a large part of a woman's aesthetic and sexual appeal. From earliest times, in all types of society, the female breast has been the focus as an object of art. Many

1

and varied have been (and still are in some societies of the world) the attempts to produce a variety of ideal breast silhouettes. In Europe in the seventeenth century and in some African tribes today, breasts have been flattened by a variety of methods for the sake of fashion. Breasts are mutilated, tattooed and jewel-hung to produce the ideal sexual image. In our day and culture, breasts are regarded more as objects of sexual arousal than the purpose for which anatomically they were originally intended—the nutrition of the infant.

Many women have mixed feelings about this 'double duty' that their breasts fulfil in our society. Within recent years there has been a welcome swing back towards breastfeeding, with all the benefits this gives to both mother and baby. Less emphasis is placed on altered breast shape, and the more natural look is in vogue.

But whatever emphasis is placed on shape and size, breasts are as prone as any other organ of the body to a variety of disease processes. It is fortunate indeed that any such disease process can be detected early by the very nature of the breasts' situation. Thus treatment of any problem stands a high chance of success if begun early enough. It should be every woman's undertaking to keep her breasts in a healthy condition and to seek medical advice if she should suspect any problem. It is hoped that this book will help all women to fulfil this task without fear, but with insight and a modicum of knowledge.

# Part 1
## The Young Breast

# ONE

# Development of the Breast, 0–20 Years

Human babies are born with two rudimentary breasts. There is no difference in size or shape between male and female at this stage. It is only later, at puberty, that the difference between the sexes becomes obvious. This difference in later development is under the control of specific hormones. In the female these hormones are responsible for the onset of ovulation and menstruation, as well as the growth of the breasts. Profound changes occur at this time of life—in awakening sexuality as well as physical changes in the reproductive system. Breast development is just one part of the overall maturation of this system.

## Faulty development of breasts

As early as the 6th week of pre-natal life the beginnings of breast development can be seen. In the tiny embryo a number of small swellings (papillae) can be seen lying along two specific lines on the front of the chest. These lines run from the armpit to the groin and are known as 'milk-ridges'. Within the next few weeks all but two of the papillae have disappeared. The two that remain are situated on the upper chest wall and it is these that will ultimately develop into the fully formed breasts of the mature woman.

As with all developmental processes, occasionally mistakes can occur, and breast development is no exception to this. The papillae along the milk-ridges can fail to disappear. This can lead to extra, or 'supernumerary', potential breasts being present at birth. This can occur at any position along the milk-ridges, from the armpit to the groin. Often no further development occurs in these extra sites, but only a small rudimentary pigmented swelling remains—rather like a mole on the skin. It is rare for fully formed milk secreting breasts to develop in these unusual sites. It is only if this happens at puberty, or if the position is one which causes irritation (such as the armpit), that surgical removal is necessary. Strangely enough this type of abnormality is seen more often in the male than the female.

On the opposite side of the coin, too much of the milk-ridge can disappear. This leads to the absence of a breast. Fortunately this is a rare condition, as there is nothing that can be done.

## The newborn breast

Newborn babies of both sexes often have some swelling in either one or both breasts. This is due to the action of their mother's hormones on this tissue. (Some baby girls also have vaginal bleeding, due to a similar cause.) Occasionally there is a whitish discharge from these swollen breasts, rather like milk. This is known as 'witch's milk'. Usually this swelling subsides spontaneously within a few days, but it may last longer if the baby is breastfed. This is again due to the action of the maternal hormones, this time being secreted in the milk.

This breast enlargement can sometimes become lumpy, red and obviously tender, but the usual course of events is for this to disappear with no treatment. Very occasionally infection will occur and need antibiotic treatment. For reassurance, mothers should get advice from their doctors or health visitors about this common condition.

## Changes at puberty

Puberty is that time of life when the secondary sex characteristics show a rate of growth which outstrips the growth that is continuing in the rest of the child's body. In boys the penis and scrotum develop and the characteristic distribution of pubic hair makes its appearance.

In girls the most obvious sign of impending womanhood is the development of the breasts. Other changes are also occurring in the girl's reproductive system; the uterus is developing and the ovaries are preparing for their monthly task of shedding an egg (ovum), or maybe more than one. This development reaches its climax with the onset of the periods, showing that reproductivity in the girl has begun. Hair is grown in both the pubic regions and in the armpits, as in boys, but in the young woman it is the development of her breasts that shows her that physical adult life is not too far away. At this time there may also be a temporary enlargement in the breasts of many boys, causing them an agony of embarrassment, but this will subside in a matter of a few months and the contours of the young man's chest will return to the masculine shape.

## Timing of puberty

This can be variable. Some girls begin breast development as early as 9 or 10 years of age and have fully developed breasts by the time they are 12 or 13 years old. (Periods in these girls often also begin at around 10 or 11 years.) But the average age at which breast development begins is around 11 to 12 years. The timing of this spurt of reproductive growth is under hormonal control. The release of these specialized hormones is under the control of a specific part of the brain known as the hypothalamus. There does seem to be a genetic inheritance at work (as indeed with all physical characteristics) in the determination of the onset of reproductive growth. Many girls will start their periods at much the same age as did their mothers a generation before—and breast development will run a similar course.

To obtain an average there must be a certain number of girls who develop secondary sexual characteristics later than the average 13 years. These girls will tend to reach full breast development by the time they are around 16 to 17 years of age—and will also start menstruating at this age. On the whole, these girls tend to be the slim, athletic types who will have small breasts throughout life.

7

## Size and shape of breasts

There is an enormous variation in the size and shape of women's breasts. In fact—along with all the other miracles of human body structure and personality—the breasts of each woman are unique to her, and her alone.

Early on in the development of the breasts at puberty, the size between the two breasts may vary quite markedly, giving rise to a 'lopsided' look which can cause worry to both the girl and her mother. But this variation in growth will even out over the succeeding months and the breasts will both be much the same size, although not exactly, when fully developed at around 16 to 17 years of age.

The base of each breast is situated on the chest wall between the 2nd and 6th ribs on each side. A small 'tail' of breast tissue extends up into the armpit in most women. (This is important to remember when it comes to examining your own breasts for lumps.) The breast tissue then protrudes to a varying degree towards the nipple area.

There is absolutely nothing that can be done to influence the size of a woman's breasts. It is probably true to say that no woman is 100 per cent happy about the size or shape of her breasts—they are either too small, too large, too pendulous and heavy or just not (to her) an ideal shape. Many are the advertisements on ways to increase your 'bust' size by exercise and various stimulatory procedures. However, exercise will only develop the muscles of the underlying chest wall on which the breasts are situated. So while it is true that the size of the breasts may appear to increase, this is merely due to the fact that they have been pushed further forward by the improved muscle tone. There is no actual increase in the amount of breast tissue. Splashing breasts with alternate hot and cold water can temporarily stimulate the blood supply to the skin of the breast, especially around the nipple area. The nipple will then stand out from the breast more definitively—as also occurs during sexual stimulation. This again can give the illusion of an increase in the breast size, but has no long-lasting effect.

Many women worry that small breasts will not be as satisfying sexually to their partners as large breasts. Concern is also frequently expressed that breastfeeding will be less effective. But both of these worries have little foundation. From the purely physical viewpoint small breasts will secrete just as adequate a supply of milk as larger breasts. From the sexual angle, it is the attitude with which women regard the sexual symbolism of their breasts which is of far more importance than the actual size or shape.

Women with heavy, pendulous breasts have probably more reason to be concerned than women with small breasts. (After all, there are many excellent bras that can give the illusion of larger breasts, but there is little that can be done to camouflage large breasts.) As well as providing great difficulties with clothes of all kinds, large breasts can be uncomfortable and heavy—particularly so in warm weather. The young girl with large breasts can go through agonies of embarrassment at school as she compares the size of her breasts with those of her friends. In extreme cases the services of a plastic surgeon will be needed to reduce the size of over-large breasts. But much thought and skilled advice must be given before embarking on such procedures. Remember, too, that overweight will cause breasts to appear larger. As well as a thicker layer of fat on the chest wall throwing the breasts forwards, there will also be an increase in the fatty tissue in the breast itself. So losing weight will have a beneficial effect on some oversized breasts, as long as the overweight problem has not existed for too long. If this is the case the connective tissue of the breasts will have become permanently stretched. Breasts under these conditions never return to an aesthetically pleasing shape without surgery. So it is better not to become overweight in the first place!

One final thing to be reviewed before proceeding to internal breast structure and function is the 'stretch marks' that can appear on the developing breast. These are similar to those that occur on the abdomen during pregnancy. They are due to the break-up of tiny pieces of elastic tissue immediately below the skin by the rapid increase in size of the breasts at puberty. Little can be done to avoid these marks apart from wearing a well-supporting bra as soon as breast development starts increasing rapidly. Preventing the weight of the breast continually pulling on the underlying tissue will reduce stretch marks to a minimum. Fortunately these tiny marks quickly fade and become almost invisible over the succeeding months.

## Mature bust structure and functions

The breast is composed of a large number of specialized glandular cells which secrete milk immediately following the birth of a baby. The milk glands are organized into 20 or so lobes, each containing many milk-producing glands, and separated from each other by a strong framework of connective tissues, vital to the support of the breast. Attachment of this strong fibrous framework is to the chest wall and to the skin of the breast, so that the shape of the breast is very much dependent on this tissue. With increasing age this connective tissue weakens and is one of the factors in the alteration of shape in the breast as the woman matures (see page 71).

Between the connective tissue framework and the actual milk-producing glands are a multitude of fat cells. It is these cells that give the breast its smooth feminine contours.

Looking at the milk-secreting glands of the breast in more detail, it can be seen that each lobe has its own milk duct which opens on the surface of the nipple (see illustration on page 11). Immediately below the opening on to the nipple, the duct is enlarged to form a collecting chamber. The milk collects here before being secreted from the nipple, and is important in the mechanics of breastfeeding (see page 57).

In addition, the breast contains blood vessels, lymph vessels and nerves—as do all other parts of the body—to ensure the correct metabolism of these organs. There are also tiny muscles associated with the milk ducts and the nipple, concerned with the expulsion of milk and the

*Section of Breast*

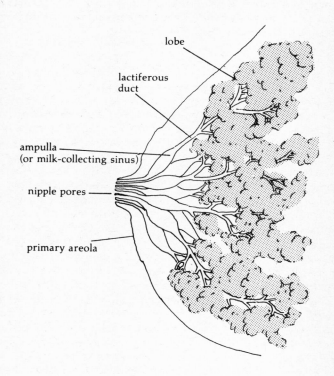

lobe

lactiferous
duct

ampulla
(or milk-collecting sinus)

nipple pores

primary areola

Adapted from *Textbook for Midwives*
by Margaret Myles (Churchill Livingstone, 1985)

11

alteration in shape of the nipple respectively. (But there is no way in which these minute muscles can be 'trimmed' by exercise to improve the size of a small breast!)

## The nipple and surrounding areola

The nipple of each breast is situated at the apex of the cone-shaped breast. This nipple itself is surrounded by an area of darker skin known as the areola. In dark-skinned women this areola is a dark brown colour, while in fair-skinned women and redheads it is a varying shade of pink. It is under this areola of the breast that the milk ducts from deep in the breast are situated before opening out on to the nipple. During pregnancy, the areola becomes darker, particularly in dark-skinned women (see page 48). Also on the areola can be seen small swellings known as Montgomery's tubercles. These are modified sweat-glands (as indeed is the whole breast) and enlarge during pregnancy and lactation. Enlargement of Montgomery's tubercles occurs early in pregnancy and continues to be prominent throughout pregnancy and breastfeeding.

As with breasts, nipples come in all sorts of shapes and sizes. Some nipples protrude from the surrounding breast tissue in a cylindrical shape all the time, while some only become so during sexual arousal, excessive cold and breastfeeding; other nipples lie flat against the areola, and yet others are inverted. (These latter will need special care during pregnancy if breastfeeding is to be successful; see page 50). The surface of the nipple can be seen to be marked with many small crevices, which are the openings of the milk ducts. In the non-active breast these crevices can contain a cheesy-like secretion. This is quite normal and should be washed gently away at bath times. Any excessive or unusual discharge from the nipple should send a woman to her doctor for his advice and any treatment that may be necessary (see page 39).

## Functions of the breast

Physiologically, the breasts are primarily intended as milk-producing organs to feed the young of the species. But today's society has decreed that this function, in many instances, is now secondary to the sexual symbolism of the breasts. Immediately after the Second World War, breast-feeding showed a marked decline. Breasts were boosted (often quite literally!) into the forefront of the 'body beautiful'. Latterly there has been an upswing in the number of women breastfeeding their babies. But breasts still remain a potent sex symbol, playing a large part in sexual attraction and love play. Shape and size is of much concern to many women in this connotation. Probably women's ideas on an 'ideal bust' are very different from the ideas of the very men they wish to attract! Much needless time, worry and money is spent on trying to alter an already attractive contour.

Anatomically and physiologically changes occur in the breast during sexual play. The nipple becomes erect, the veins on the breast become more prominent and the whole breast swells. In some women this is followed by a faint red flush all over the skin of the breast, associated with the swelling of the areola. At this time too, Montgomery's tubercles stand out markedly. Following orgasm, all these changes regress leaving the breast in its pre-excitation state, but in some women excessively tender. Obviously, no two women react in the same way to sexual breast play. Some women enjoy this aspect of lovemaking more than others and it is up to each couple to discover what is the most pleasing to their partner.

Breastfeeding produces similar sensual feelings in many women, as does preliminary love play. While to some women this is a bonus of breastfeeding, to others it is a cause for concern and feelings of guilt. But there is absolutely no reason why breastfeeding should not be a pleasurable sensual experience—as well as a beautifully adapted mechanism for nurturing babies. If this aspect of breastfeeding is sympathetically and clearly explained to

13

young mothers embarking on breastfeeding their babies, perhaps more women would persist in this ideal way of feeding their new sons and daughters (for breastfeeding practices, see chapter 7.

# TWO

# Bras and their Function

Bras are an integral part of the wardrobe of most women these days, but this was not always so. In fact it is only during this century that bras (or brassières to give the full name) in their present form became widely available. In ancient Greece and Rome clothes were loosely draped. Female figures were neither hidden nor enhanced. This mode of dress persisted until the sixteenth century when corsets—made with rigid, unyielding whalebone—became fashionable. These fearsome garments encased women's bodies from shoulder to hips and successfully hid the natural figure. During Regency times, when slim, tight-fitting dresses were in fashion, the 'bust' became a necessity, and 'false bosoms' were all the rage for a short time. In Victorian days the corset—again made from a variety of hard, unyielding materials—became the vogue. Bodies were squeezed and pulled into contorted shapes by these vindictive undergarments as fashion dictated. No doubt many of the 'vapours' suffered by the Victorian miss were due to her inability to breathe, eat or circulate her blood adequately! But towards the end of the nineteenth century there was a national movement to end these excesses in women's dress. Tight-lacing corsetry was frowned on, and the garments previously worn were replaced by a firm bodice of lighter, more pliable material.

It was the First World War that brought about the revolution in women's undergarments, paving the way for the modern bra. During these four critical years, when women were working alongside men more than ever before, they found they needed full freedom of movement. After the war, as the emancipation movement gained momentum, and 'votes for women' became eminently newsworthy, figures of a more masculine appearance were all the fashion. To aid this concept, bodices became breast-flatteners. As time went on, manufacturers realized the commercial possibilities of the bra and proceeded to exploit the fashion which was veering towards the more modern female silhouette. Bras with different cup sizes were produced after research into the actual differences in women's bust shapes and sizes. This market expanded rapidly until it became the multi-million pound business it is in the western world today.

These changes in fashion were mirrored—to a greater or lesser extent—in most of the western world. In other parts of the world, fashions, born of necessity, are obviously very different, and many women have never worn, and will never wear, a bra during their whole lifespan.

## To wear, or not to wear, a bra

What are the reasons for wearing a bra at all? Are these based on good sound commonsense, or is it just a dictate of fashion that makes women fold themselves daily into a bra? Obviously *fashion* plays a large part, and women are much influenced by the vast amount of advertising material to be found in all aspects of the media. Silhouettes change with fashion, and so does the need for different bras. In fact, most women have a number of bras in their wardrobes to accommodate both their day and evening needs.

Another reason is *comfort*. Most women will find wearing a bra more comfortable than going braless, and particularly so if they have large, heavy breasts. Women with smaller breasts may not be so aware of this aspect. But they also will probably feel the need for a bra—to enhance their bust-line. Bras with extra padding to boost a small bust are readily available (see page 19). These bras have great value in boosting a small-breasted woman's figure to the standard fitting dresses and sweaters.

During lactation, a specially adapted bra (see page 62) may well be more comfortable. At this time, breasts are full and heavy and the support given by a well-fitting bra will reduce subsequent sagging of the breast due to stretching of supporting tissues. Milk production will not be affected whether or not a bra is worn.

A well-fitting bra, worn regularly, will reduce to a minimum the stretching of the tissue supporting the breast. This is of especial importance during the early years of active development of the breast, as well as during lactation. Later on in life, following the menopause when the subcutaneous fat of the breast is reduced, a well-fitting bra can help prevent sagging of the mature breast.

So while the wearing of a bra has no beneficial effect on the physiological function of the breast (in other words, milk production) there are aesthetic and comfort aspects in the routine wearing of this type of undergarment. Nowadays, however, many younger women do find it more comfortable not to wear a bra in hot weather. And present-day fashion favours the 'natural' look with soft, light bras.

### At what age should a bra start to be worn?

As has been seen above, there is no absolute necessity to wear a bra at all from the physiological point of view. Similarly there is also no absolute rule as to when a young girl should buy her first bra. Theoretically a light support is a good idea as soon as the breast tissue is sufficient to become noticeable when the girl runs or jumps. But, practically, a bra will probably be bought when the girl's peers are also purchasing a bra!

Fortunately, theoretical and practical aspects usually coincide and most girls are wearing bras by the time they are 13 years old.

### Types of bra

Before discussing the types of bra available, it is a good idea to consider just what the average woman requires from her bra.

- It should be comfortable
- It should give her the silhouette she wishes

- It should wash well and easily
- Straps should ideally be adaptable to suit a variety of dress styles and not cut into shoulders
- There should be no obvious—or uncomfortable—rigid supports or seams
- There should be an adequate range of types, sizes and colours from which to choose

With the wide range of styles and sizes on the market, most women are able to find a bra to suit their requirements, although this may take several years of trial and error. It is all too easy, when young, to choose a glamorous lacy bra only to find when you get it home that the fit and comfort leave much to be desired. Eventually most women will settle on one particular style and size for everyday wear, with probably one or two extra, more exciting bras for wear on special occasions.

Bras could be classified in any number of ways. But the following differing types will encompass most of the styles available.

*Strapless or with straps*
*Strapless bras* are best suited to those women with small breasts. Larger, heavier breasts will need to be supported by a strap over the shoulders. To be of any value in helping to produce a rounded silhouette, a strapless bra must have some degree of wiring beneath the cup. Unless the bra fits well, this can be extremely uncomfortable. Incidentally, there is no truth in the comment that wired bras are a factor in the causation of cancer of the breast. Any ill-fitting bra—and this includes those strapless bras with wired cups—can, by constant friction, cause a fibrous thickening in the breast tissue. On changing the bra, this thickening will disappear within a few months. If this is not the case, medical advice should be sought.

Soft, strapless bras are a useful asset under sun and beachwear. These tend to flatten the breasts, but are worn by many women under these circumstances for the sake of comfort.

*Strapped bras* should ideally have wide enough straps to ensure that there is no cutting into the shoulders. Elasticated straps are the most suitable, particularly for the larger-sized bras where several pounds of breast weight have to be supported throughout a long day.

Strapped bras should also ideally be versatile in the position of the straps. This will ensure that a favourite bra can be worn with a variety of dress styles.

### Padded or unpadded bras

Padded bras are obviously for those women who have small breasts, but wish to add a few centimetres to their bust measurement. This is both for appearance sake and also to ensure a better fit on the many garments that are made for women with a standard, larger bust. The padding is usually confined to the under-bust part of the bra. It must be safe, comfortable and should not ruckle with wear.

Both padded and unpadded bras are made in a variety of materials—cotton and various synthetic fibres being the two main types. Cotton bras tend to keep their colour better through numerous washings than those made from synthetic fibres—but possibly the appearance of a lacy nylon bra has more feminine appeal?

### Back or front-fastening bras

Most women—with two main exceptions—seem to prefer a back-fastening bra (although many women will adjust the fastening on the bra at the front, and then slide the bra round!). But there are two aspects of a woman's life where front-fastening bras are more popular and suitable. During lactation, when breasts are heavier, front-fastening bras are very much more convenient; most nursing bras fasten at the front (see page 62). Similarly, women suffering from conditions such as various rheumatic diseases, for example, will often find a front-fastening bra easier to wear and fasten.

All types of bra are available with a varying width of band below the 'cup' part of the bra. Slim women will require the minimum width in this position. But those women with extra weight in this part of their body will find a deeper bra more comfortable, as well as helping to control their figures.

These then are the main types of bra available. There are other specialized bras which are necessary for use under special conditions—for example, during breastfeeding (see page 62) and following a mastectomy (see page 95).

## How to buy your bra

Ideally, you should try on any bra before you buy. Also, the help of a trained corsetière is helpful. But in reality these skilled ladies are hard to find, and most of us buy our bras from one or other of the main self-service stores. Usually, after a few mistakes, the right size and style is found and similar replacements bought when necessary. An idea of your correct size is a 'must' if you are buying your bra from these stores. To determine your correct size, you need to take two measurements into account. Firstly, the measurement around your chest *below* your breasts, will give you the actual bra size you should buy. Secondly, the cup size will depend on the size of your breasts: if you have small breasts, cup 'A' is for you; similarly, cup 'D' is for you if you have heavy, pendulous breasts; cup sizes 'B' and 'C' fit the majority of women and here it is very much a matter of trial and error as to which you will need. Remember that it is unwise to try on and buy a bra immediately before a period. Many women's breasts swell for a few days immediately prior to a period, due to water retention. So if, for example, you decide you need a 'C' cup at this time, the chances are high that this will be too large for the first three weeks of your menstrual cycle. Perhaps one extra—larger—bra for wear during these few days would be a good idea?

It is worth taking a little time and thought over the purchase of your bra.

A well-fitting bra, as well as being comfortable, will alter the appearance of the clothes you wear. Remember bras are worn, on average, for around 18 hours out of every 24, and this is a long time in which to feel uncomfortable. Some women with very heavy breasts, or perhaps also during the latter weeks of pregnancy, will find it more comfortable to wear a bra throughout the 24 hours. Under these circumstances it is especially important that the bra fits well.

## 'Topless'

We have seen that from a physiological viewpoint a bra is unnecessary and, anatomically, the wearing of a bra will only put off the day when the firm elasticity of the breast tissues begins to sag. So it is for comfort and aesthetic considerations that bras are worn. But what about the growing trend in the west for women to go around without any covering over their breasts when sunbathing in warm weather? Leaving aesthetic considerations aside, are there any problems associated with this practice?

In many parts of the tropical world, it is the custom for women's breasts to be bare and certainly no harm comes to them. Fair-skinned European women may have some initial problems of sunburn of the skin of the breast and particularly on the delicate tissue surrounding the nipple. But the usual care on time of exposure to the sun and adequate application of sun-screen products should reduce this problem to a minimum. Active sports in the sun will probably be uncomfortable 'topless' unless the breasts are very small. So many women who sunbathe topless will be reaching for their bras as soon as any active pursuits are contemplated.

# THREE

# Problems in the Young Breast

Although there are few problems in the young breast, there are one or two conditions that may cause concern. This chapter discusses such problems, and describes the required treatment and measures for prevention.

## 'Jogger's nipple'

Yes, it really is a well-known diagnosis—for men as well as women. One only has to watch the regular up-and-down movement of a T-shirt over the chest in those energetic joggers who pound our streets day and night to understand why the poor old nipple reacts, at times strongly, to this treatment. With each forward step, arms and shoulders swing across, rubbing the material of the T-shirt or sweater on the delicate tissue of the nipple. As well as consisting of especially delicate tissue, the nipple, standing out from the surrounding tissue as it does, receives the full force of the up-and-down movement. The top layer of skin becomes rubbed off, leaving the exquisitely tender tissue beneath to receive the full force of the continuing trauma. (Marathon runners have been known to arrive at their destination with bleeding nipples.)

*Treatment for 'jogger's nipple'*

1 Avoid further trauma until healing is complete.
2 Bathe with sodium bicarbonate solution.
3 Smear with antiseptic cream to prevent infection, or smear with antibiotic cream (obtainable on prescription) if infection has already occurred.

1 Stop jogging! (Try walking instead).
2 Men can jog in summer with no upper covering, but women should wear a well-fitting bra.
3 When sweaters must be worn in winter, apply a gauze dressing stuck down firmly over nipple area.

'Jogger's nipple' is a self-inflicted injury, maybe, but nevertheless one which causes much needless discomfort. With a little forethought this condition need never occur.

## Pain associated with menstruation

The onset of menstruation in the teenage girl announces the arrival of physical maturity. Breast development will usually be well advanced by the time the first period occurs. It is at this stage the young woman may first experience breast pain. This is very common in many women, the pain occurring only during the few days immediately prior to the period. The breasts are tender to any mild trauma, and some girls find sport a problem at this time of the month. The cause of this pain is due to the excess fluid held in the body—and this includes the breast tissue—during the latter part of the menstrual cycle. As soon as the period begins, these unpleasant sensations disappear. Little can be done to relieve the pain and tenderness, except to give aspirin or paracetamol compounds at regular intervals. A well-fitting bra will support the breast and make the girl feel more comfortable. A few girls have such severe pain and tenderness as to make this an excuse for avoiding school sports. (For other causes of breast pain, see page 35—pain in the breast is more common in the 20–50 age group.)

## Breast lumps in adolescence

*Fibroadenoma*
There are only two types of breast lumps that are at all common under the age of 20 years. The first is a swelling

known as a fibroadenoma. This lump can occur in any part of the breast, and, being painless, is usually discovered quite accidentally by the girl as she showers or bathes. There may be more than one of these swellings in the breast. These lumps consist of a conglomeration of breast and fibrous tissue. They are difficult to pin down exactly in any one part of the breast. The lump is quite firm to the touch, but 'runs away' from examining fingers. Medical advice should be sought to make a certain diagnosis. Most surgeons will remove this type of distinctive swelling, not because it is malignant, but because it can grow into a fair-sized swelling and thus deform the developing breast tissue. This operation is quick, and a day or two in hospital only is required. A hairline scar is all that will be left as a reminder of the breast swelling.

*Fibrocystic disease*
Fibrocystic disease of the breasts is the other common cause of lumps in the breasts of young women. This is a condition where there is a multitude of small, distinct swellings all over the breast. Frequently both breasts are simultaneously affected. The lumps are tender to the touch, and become more obvious and painful immediately prior to a period. In fact, fibrocystic disease of the breast is closely allied to hormone levels in the body. At adolescence, these levels (oestrogen in particular) have not as yet become stabilized. So fibrocystic swellings can vary from week to week. As a girl matures, and her hormone levels settle into a regular pattern, these swellings in her breasts will often disappear altogether. But in a number of women the fibrocystic disease will develop further (see page 37 for details.)

However, as with all swellings in the breast, it is advisable for the young woman with possible early fibrocystic disease to contact her doctor to be sure of the diagnosis. At this stage, no treatment will be necessary other than routine measures such as a well-fitting bra, and aspirin to help the pain if this is a problem in the days immediately before a period.

## Hygiene

Hygiene is an important part of breast care. Along with other parts of the body, the breasts should be washed regularly and dried thoroughly. This latter is particularly important for women with large, heavy breasts. In hot weather especially, the skin under heavy breasts can become red and sore unless particular care is taken. A light dusting of talc in this area is often beneficial. But be sure to dry the skin thoroughly first, or you will be compounding the problem with a sticky mass of excess talc adhering to the skin.

There can normally be a small amount of secretion from the nipples, which can become caked on the skin in this situation. This should be gently washed away and, again, the nipple area thoroughly dried. (Any excessive, watery or blood-stained discharge from the nipple *must* be reported *immediately* to your doctor; see page 39.)

Sore places on the skin of the breast can arise from an ill-fitting bra. The obvious remedy for this is to buy another bra and this time, to be sure you get a correct fit, try on a bra until you find a style and size that suit you. Treatment for any sore spots due to this cause is by an antiseptic cream and scrupulous hygiene.

*Part 2*
*The 'Active' Breast*

# Introduction: the Years Between 20 and 40

Broadly speaking, the years between 20 and 40 are the years of child-bearing for most women. Of course, reproductive life can start earlier than this and continue later. But most women will complete their families during these years, so it is at this time that the breasts are active. With each pregnancy changes occur and milk is produced following delivery of the baby. Even if, for one reason or another, breastfeeding is not established, the changes for this physiological function still occur in the breasts.

With all the activity due to pregnancy in the breast at this time in a woman's life, as well as the usual cyclical changes due to the regular menstrual periods, it is advisable that all women should be aware of the possible problems that can arise in their breasts. Regular, routine examination of the breast to detect early signs of problems is an excellent habit to acquire early in these reproductive years.

This section begins with an explanation of how women can perform a regular monthly examination of their breasts—what they may find—and what to do if they do discover any abnormality (Chapter 4). Abnormal conditions which can affect the breast are then discussed, together with the treatment necessary (Chapter 5). Cancer of the breast can occur in this age group, but it is more common—along with most other cancers—in the over-40 age group. So for this particular abnormality of the breast, Part 3 (particularly Chapter 10) should be consulted.

Finally, the normal changes occurring in the breast during pregnancy are described, together with a discussion on breastfeeding (Chapters 6 and 7).

# FOUR

# Self-Examination of Breasts

It may seem an obvious thing to say, but *you* will be the first person in all probability to discover a lump in your breast. After all, you are the one that knows your body best. And, as you bath or shower it will be *your* fingers that come across the unusual swelling in the normally smooth curve of your breast. For many women this is a surprise happening. By the time the lump has become this obvious, chances are that it has been there for some considerable time. And if the lump should be a cancer (*but do remember that about 80 per cent of all lumps in the breast are due to causes other than cancer*), valuable time has been lost before starting treatment. So the sensible course to pursue is to examine your breasts regularly, at specified intervals. In this way the smallest abnormality will be found and active steps for treatment can be started early.

## Timing of self-examination session

It is important to undertake this 'self-help' action at regular intervals. For women who menstruate regularly, the last day or so of the menstrual period is the best time to do this. If the breasts are examined immediately before a period is due, or during the first day or two of bleeding, the breasts will, in many women, feel frighteningly 'lumpy'. This is due to the effects of circulating hormones in the body at this time affecting the breast tissue. But, as menstruation begins, hormonal levels change and breasts once more assume their smooth contours. Any lump felt at this time should receive *immediate* medical attention.

Set aside ten minutes every month to do this test. Perhaps before you take your bath or shower at night, or maybe during the course of a quiet afternoon when all the

## Breast examination chart

| | 19— | 19— | 19— |
|---|---|---|---|
| January | | | |
| February | | | |
| March | | | |
| April | | | |
| May | | | |
| June | | | |
| July | | | |
| August | | | |
| September | | | |
| October | | | |
| November | | | |
| December | | | |

family are 'napping' if young, or at school if older, will suit your routine best. But whenever you decide will be most convenient, do keep it up. Perhaps mark off in your diary when you last checked your breasts or keep a simple chart, such as shown on page 31, so that you can easily see when your next self-examination is due. Fill in the actual date when you last examined your breasts.

Women who menstruate irregularly should endeavour to examine their breasts at least every six weeks, choosing a time when they have just finished menstruating.

Remember, if you have a family, you owe it to them as well as yourself to keep fit and healthy—and this means getting *early* treatment for any problem that may arise.

## How to examine your own breasts

*Step 1* (see illustrations opposite).
1 Sit in front of your mirror stripped to the waist.
2 Look at your breasts

  - do you notice anything different from usual?
  - any change in contour?
  - any pulling of the nipple to one side?
  - any discharge from the nipple?

3 Raise your arms and put your hands behind your head; recheck on above points.

*Step 2* (see illustrations opposite).
1 Lie on your back on your bed with a pillow under one shoulder. (This will throw the breast you are about to examine forward and so make any swelling more obvious.)
2 In your 'mind's eye' divide your breast into four quarters.
3 With the *flat* of your hand (never use finger and thumb—you will automatically feel lumps everywhere as you pinch up the breast tissue) feel gently, but firmly, each quarter of your breast.

32

**Step 1**

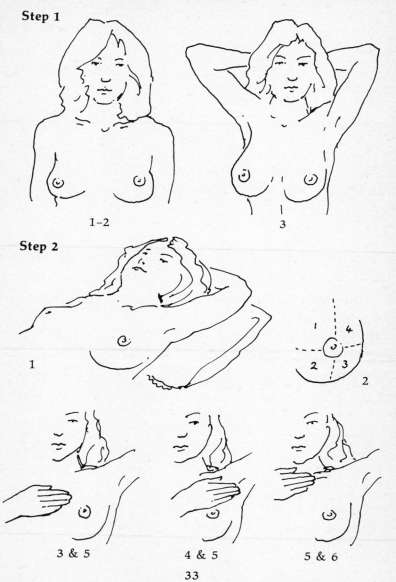

1–2                           3

**Step 2**

1

2

3 & 5          4 & 5          5 & 6

4 Feel up into your armpit; your breast tissue extends in a 'tail' up here, and so must receive your attention.
5 Repeat with the other breast, remembering to move the pillow to under the other shoulder.
6 Finally, check that there are no lumps or swellings in either armpit or immediately along your collar-bone on either side.

Alternatively, the breast can be felt in a circular fashion starting at the nipple and radiating out in ever-increasing circles. Choose whichever method you find most comfortable.

Ten minutes is a generous allowance of time to perform this simple test—and surely you owe it to yourself and your family to take this time out of a busy schedule once a month?

But supposing all your worst fears are realized and you think you feel a lump. First of all—*don't panic!* The chances are high that it is *not* a cancerous lump. Then—check again. And if you are sure that you can feel something unusual in the breast tissue, telephone your doctor for an early appointment. No need to rush down to the surgery and demand to be seen that very minute. But be sure you do see your doctor within the next three or four days. His experienced fingers will be able to tell you straightaway if the lump is likely to be a sinister one or not. If he is in any doubt, he will send you off with an early appointment to see a specialist.

But whatever the outcome, you have done your part in ensuring that the appropriate treatment for whatever is causing your particular swelling is given early.

FIVE

# Problems in the Active Breast

As breasts become 'active', there is more chance of problems occurring—but these are by no means always serious. In this chapter, I describe problems associated with the active breast and how to deal with them.

## Pain in the breast

*Due to injury*
This is the most obvious cause of breast pain. It is indeed surprising that breasts do not receive more bumps and blows than other parts of the body. One would have thought the very situation and size of this part of the body would have made this form of injury a commonplace event. The reason why this is not so is that women automatically protect their breasts, either with their hands or by avoiding obvious traumas. This is, of course, especially so when the breasts are tender premenstrually. Probably the most common causes of blows to the breast are found during the years when there are small children around the house. The fury of a young toddler in a temper tantrum does not respect the tenderness of his mother's breast as he lands out thumps and blows in all directions. Ill-fitting car seat-belts can also rub tender breasts and cause considerable pain. Under these circumstances, try to either change the type of seat-belt or to adjust your existing one.

Blows to the breast are extremely painful and cause women much concern as to possible long-term effects. A tender lump can result from a blow. This is due to bruising (that is, leakage of blood from fracture of tiny blood vessels) in the breast tissue. This heals slowly and usually the breast tissue returns to normality, with no long-term effects. Occasionally, a hard fibrous swelling may be left.

This can feel very similar to a cancerous lump and under these circumstances you should most certainly seek your doctor's advice (see Chapter 10—cancer of the breast).

But does a blow on the breast of itself produce a cancer? This is the question about which many women are concerned. Blows themselves do not cause cancer. But if a lump persists for several weeks following a blow, medical advice should be sought. The lump may be due to the normal healing process, as described above, or it may be that the blow has highlighted an existing lump, which must be further investigated. So the message is to seek medical advice early if you have a persistent lump in your breast following an injury.

Injury to the breast can also occur through over-vigorous lovemaking. But this form of trauma is usually limited by the sensitivity of the breasts. Such trauma heals quickly and completely.

During breastfeeding nipples can become cracked and sore and this is a common cause of breast pain—along with enlarged breasts—at this time of life (see Chapter 7).

*Pain associated with menstruation*
This is such a commonplace occurrence that it can almost be termed a normal phenomenon. As mentioned previously, sensations of acute tenderness are due to the water retention that occurs in the body at this time. Little can be done to relieve this tenderness except to take pain-killing drugs if the pain is especially troublesome. Possibly some women may find reducing their fluid intake slightly for the week immediately preceding their period helpful. Fortunately this form of breast pain is self-limiting because, with the onset of menstruation, these feelings of tenderness will disappear.

There is a further form of breast pain, however, that occurs on a regular basis associated with the menstrual cycle. Again, the pain can be severe immediately prior to the onset of the period. This can be distinguished from the more usual type of premenstrual breast tenderness in three ways:

1 It is 'pain' rather than 'tenderness' that is the problem, affecting usually both breasts.
2 This pain is more pronounced and lasts longer—up to two or three weeks of the menstrual cycle—than premenstrual tenderness.
3 The breasts feel nodular.

This type of pain can be due to *fibrocystic disease* (see page 24) and is thought to be related to the level of certain hormones—oestrogen in particular—in the blood. ('Mastitis' or 'cystic disease of the breast' are other terms used for the condition.) It is a common condition of the breast—about one in five women suffer from this at some time during their reproductive years. It is *not* a cancerous condition. But it is important that any lumps in the breast should receive medical advice. So do check with your doctor if your breasts are lumpy and painful for a large part of your menstrual cycle. As the name implies, fibrocystic disease of the breast can lead on to formation of cysts in the breast tissue, where one or more of the nodular swellings becomes filled with fluid. This can happen quickly, and be associated with a sudden sharp pain in the breast. The swelling thus formed will feel rubbery to the touch and slides away from your fingers as you examine this new phenomenon. Depending on where this cystic swelling is situated, there may be an associated discharge from the nipple.

Your doctor will probably wish to refer you to a surgeon who specializes in breast lumps if you have a cystic condition in the breast. Treatment will be either aspiration of the cyst (involving removal of the fluid in the cyst with a syringe) or removal of the cyst surgically under a general anaesthetic. Many surgeons prefer to pursue the latter course in order to be quite sure that the cyst is not a manifestation of an underlying cancerous lump. But whatever treatment is given, do be reassured that the surgeon dealing with breast problems has vast experience. Sensitive, experienced fingers will be able to detect, with great accuracy, the cause of your particular swelling. Your part in this procedure must be to make the initial contact with your doctor. Do not be afraid or shy to do this. Every doctor would far rather reassure you on an insignificant lump in the breast rather than miss a potentially serious one. And do remember again that the majority of lumps in the breast are *not* due to cancer. Remember also that cancerous lumps in the breast stand a good chance of complete cure if treatment commences early enough.

While discussing conditions of the breast associated with hormone levels, many women are concerned regarding any possible effects that the contraceptive pill may have on their breasts. Recent research has shown that women who have taken the contraceptive pill for a number of years tend to suffer less from such conditions as fibrocystic disease of the breast than do women who use other forms of contraception. Also there appears to be no related link between use of the contraceptive pill and cancer of the breast.

*Other causes*

1 An ill-fitting, or too tight bra can cause pain in the breast. But by the time this age group is reached, most women will have settled to one particular type of bra which suits them and is comfortable. But it is as well to check the fit of your bra, particularly if you have put on weight recently.
2 Cold weather can cause quite severe pain in some women's breasts. The obvious answer to this is to wear warmer clothing.
3 Conditions affecting the tissues of the chest wall causing pain can seem to be related to the breast. Any strain which affects the muscles of the chest wall underlying the breast tissue is one example of this. Occasionally, the joints between the ribs and the breastbone can become painful, and this type of pain (sometimes severe and of a lengthy duration) can also seem to radiate to the breast tissue. For both these conditions pain-killing drugs are of value, together with avoidance of any strenuous activities that have been noted to bring on the pain.

Pain in the breast is an uncomfortable and unpleasant symptom. As has been seen it can be due to any one of a number of causes. A visit to your doctor, for diagnosis and treatment, should be your course of action for any persistent and/or recurrent pain in the breasts.

## Discharge from the nipples

This is a symptom about which you should *always* consult your doctor. There are a number of causes of nipple discharge—most causes being trivial and easily treated, but a few are more serious, requiring early and urgent attention.

*Discharges which are not serious*
First of all, two common discharges from the nipple which need cause you no worry. First, and obviously, is the production of milk from both nipples on the third day following the birth of a baby. This will have been preceded —both intermittently in the latter weeks of pregnancy and continuously after the birth of the baby—by the secretion of a thin, watery fluid known as 'colostrum' (see Chapter 7). Secondly, the vast majority of nipples continuously secrete a little fluid. This normally evaporates and is rubbed off on clothing. But occasionally, the secretion dries and is obvious either as a soft cheesy lump on the surface of the nipple or as a stain on clothing. Nothing further than scrupulous hygiene needs to be done. Both these types of secretion affect both nipples.

A further cause of nipple discharge that affects both breasts is that due to the taking of certain drugs. The contraceptive pill, some anti-depressant and anti-hypertensive drugs are the ones most usually involved in this form of milky discharge. These drugs all act by stimulation of the hormonal mechanism which causes milk production. This production of a milky discharge can also occur in men taking these drugs—a side-effect that can cause much embarrassment to the unfortunate sufferer. On stopping, or changing the drug (on your doctor's advice of course) this abnormal nipple discharge will cease in a week or two. Other appropriate drugs will need to be given which do not produce this unwanted side-effect.

One further type of discharge affecting both breasts can occur in women at, or near, the menopause. This is a greyish, cloudy discharge which is again closely related to the hormonal changes taking place in the body at this time of life.

*Discharges which must receive immediate advice*
While you will be wise to contact your doctor if you are worried about a discharge from your nipples that follows any of the patterns discussed above, it is vital that medical advice is sought if the discharge:

1  is from one nipple only;
2  is associated with a lump in the breast;
3  is blood-stained; or
4  is thin, watery and from one breast only.

*Discharge from one nipple associated with a lump*
This set of symptoms must receive immediate medical attention. *Cancer* of the breast is a possibility even in the under-40 age group (for further discussion, see Part 3, particularly Chapter 10).

A further cause of discharge from one nipple in this age group is due to a condition known as *duct ectasia*. Some of the milk ducts dilate and become full of the products of tissue breakdown. This produces the typical sticky discharge which ranges from a yellowish to a frankly blood-stained colour. Many women also find that their breasts become reddened and itchy around the areola. With further progression of the condition, a firm swelling may appear beneath the areola. This is due to the fibrosis of the tissues around the dilated duct. Medical advice must be sought under these circumstances (discharge associated with a 'lump'). In the early stage of duct ectasia, treatment with oestrogens will clear the condition. If the disease has progressed, surgery may be necessary to relieve the symptoms, but this condition is *not* considered to be a pre-cancerous one. Duct ectasia usually affects women in the latter end of this age group, and can also occur in menopausal women.

### Blood-stained discharge

Again, this type of nipple discharge *must* receive medical advice. There are several conditions other than *cancer* which give rise to a bloodstained discharge. But it is vitally important that a malignant growth is excluded. As we have seen, a long-standing duct ectasia can cause a blood-stained discharge. A condition known as a *intra-duct papilloma* can also give rise to this symptom. This is a benign growth in one of the milk ducts. It is usually so small that no lump is palpable in the breast. It is only when pressure of the affected part of the breast produces the typical discharge from the nipple that this form of growth is suspected. Although the vast majority of these types of growth are not cancerous, they can become so at a later date. So an operation is advised to remove the growth in the milk duct. With a simple intra-duct papilloma, the incision will be small, and practically invisible after a few months, and the breast will not be deformed in any way. Regular check-ups following this form of surgery are necessary, as women who have had one intra-duct papilloma are more likely to have further similar problems. Very occasionally, a mastectomy will be necessary if, on microscopic examination, the papilloma is found to contain cancerous cells.

*Fibrocystic disease* in its cystic phase (see page 42) can also give rise to a brownish, maybe blood-stained discharge. The cysts can be felt in the breast, and here again medical advice must be sought. Treatment will be either by aspiration of the fluid in the cyst with a syringe, or by surgical removal of the cyst.

Finally, a blood-stained discharge can occur *during pregnancy*. This requires no treatment if there is no associated breast lump. This form of discharge will cease after the birth of the baby.

*Thin watery discharge*

This type of discharge from one nipple only should receive *immediate* medical advice. It is often a sign of an underlying cancerous condition, although the actual swelling of the growth may not be large enough to be felt.

Nipple discharge is a common symptom. Unless due to obvious causes, such as milk production after pregnancy, it must always be taken seriously, and medical advice sought. But do remember that there are many causes for this symptom which have a ready solution. And remember also that if there is a cancer of the breast this is curable if diagnosed and treated early.

## Lump in the breast

In this section, non-cancerous or benign lumps in the breast will be discussed. While cancer of the breast is certainly not unknown in women below the age of 40, it is less likely to be the cause for a lump in the breast than if a lump is found in women of over 40 (see Chapter 10). That is not to say, of course, that a lump in the breast of a woman under 40 should be ignored. *Never ignore a lump in your breast—at whatever age you discover this.* Always check with your doctor, so that the cause of your particular lump can be diagnosed. And remember that around 80 per cent of all breast lumps are benign—and at the risk of being repetitive, remember too that breast cancer, if diagnosed and treated early, can be cured.

## Causes of benign lumps in the breast

*Fibrocystic disease (or mastitis)*

As was seen in Part 1 on the young breast, fibrocystic disease can cause problems very early on in life. The young girl who has just begun to menstruate regularly will feel her breasts tender and 'lumpy' particularly just before a period is due. As her hormone levels alter these symptoms will pass. But in the older, 30–40 age group, the swellings (maybe several in each breast) will persist. As you do your routine self-examination of your breasts you will feel small swellings, rather like peas under the skin, if you have fibrocystic disease. It is when one or more of the swellings become surrounded by fibrous tissue that a definite lump can be felt. This can be difficult to distinguish from a cancerous lump, and certainly one which must receive your doctor's advice. A further manifestation in fibrocystic disease of the breast is the formation of cysts in the breast tissue. These again will be definite lumps in the breast. But the texture of these will be softer, and have a rubbery feel. To get an idea of what a cystic swelling feels like, shut your eyes and move your finger gently over your eyeball.

Associated with this stage of fibrocystic disease may be a discharge from the nipple (see page 80). Occasionally there may be a sudden stabbing pain in the breast as a cyst is being formed. This is due to the stretching of the breast tissue with its integral nerve supply by the fluid under pressure in the cyst. It may be the first time you notice the typical rubbery swelling as you feel your breast after this type of pain.

*Treatment.* Once it has been firmly established that fibrocystic disease is the cause of your particular swelling (a *biopsy*, or removal of a small part of the lump, may be necessary to do this; see page 88), there are a number of treatments that can be tried to relieve the discomfort of this condition.

1 Simple treatment such as a well-fitting bra, and pain-killers at the time in the menstrual cycle when breasts are most tender, may be all that is needed.
2 Occasionally, drugs which reduce the level of water retention in the body can be useful. These are best taken immediately before a period is due.
3 Removal of the fluid content of the cyst with a syringe; this can be done under a local anaesthetic.
4 Surgical removal of the lump, under a general anaesthetic; it may be necessary to follow this line to be completely sure that the lump is benign.

Fibrocystic disease of the breast is a common condition affecting around one in five women during their reproductive years. While it is a benign condition, medical advice should always be sought, as a cancerous lump can co-exist alongside fibrocystic disease. And just because one lump proved to be due to fibrocystic disease in the past, never ignore a further lump—it could just be something more sinister.

### Fibroadenoma

These firm, well-defined lumps in the breast are the next commonest cause of swellings in the 20–40 age group. They are composed of both glandular and fibrous tissue. They grow very slowly, but can become quite large if left without treatment. They are not thought to ever become cancerous. Fibroadenoma, to experienced fingers, have a very specific feel and most doctors will be able to diagnose these lumps accurately.

*Treatment*. The treatment of fibroadenoma is removal of the lump surgically under general anaesthetic. This is done both to establish the diagnosis definitely, and also to prevent distortion of the breast tissue by a large swelling. The stay in hospital will be short, and the scar where the swelling was removed will fade to become almost invisible within a few months.

### Lipoma

A lipoma is a fatty lump. It can occur anywhere in the body, and the breast is no exception. In fact, as the breast is largely composed of fatty tissue, it is not unusual for this type of lump to occur here. It is again a benign lump.

*Treatment*. Unless the lipoma is very small, it is best removed surgically. As it continues to grow it can distort the surrounding breast tissue. Again, only a short stay in hospital is necessary, with just minimal scarring to show that a lump has been removed.

These then are the common swellings and lumps to be found in the breast. They make up for around 80 per cent of all breast swellings and are essentially benign. But *all* lumps should be checked out by your doctor and this also means each *new* lump that appears.

## The contraceptive pill and breast conditions

The years between 20 and 40 are the reproductive years for the majority of women. Hand in hand with this is the fact that these are also the years when many women take the oral contraceptive pill. And the question has doubtless crossed many women's minds whether this long-term taking of the pill can have any deleterious effects on the breast.

The pill is basically a mixture of two hormones found naturally in the body. These are given, in a range of different forms, for a specific length of time in each menstrual cycle. This effectively stops the release of an ovum from the ovary, which occurs usually around half way through each menstrual cycle. The breasts, being intimately connected with these cyclical hormonal changes, must also be affected by this artificial hormonal picture. (This artificially produced hormonal situation is similar to that which arose when pregnancy followed pregnancy in quick succession in the days before contraception became so sophisticated.)

There has never been any suggestion that prolonged taking of oral contraceptives causes a higher incidence of breast cancer. The contraceptive pill, in all its many forms, is probably the most researched medicant on the market. Had there been any connection between an increase in breast cancer and oral contraceptives, the Committee on the Safety of Drugs would have issued warnings many years ago. But several research projects have shown that women taking long-term oral contraceptives suffer less from benign breast disease. This is particularly so in the case of fibrocystic disease of the breast and fibroadenoma. So it would appear that the pill in some way *protects* against these common benign—but nevertheless worrying—breast conditions.

## Hair on the breast

This is not exactly a 'disease' of the breast, but nevertheless one which can cause some women a good deal of distress. Occasionally long hairs grow on the breast, particularly around the nipple area. These can be very noticeable, particularly in dark-skinned women.

Treatment consists of applying the usual methods of hair removal—depilatory creams, shaving or simply pulling out the longer, more obvious hairs. With all these methods, however, the hairs will return again within a few weeks. Electrolysis, in which the actual hair follicles are destroyed by a minute electric current, is the only permanent answer to the problem. This is a skilled treatment and you should seek advice from someone specializing in this form of treatment if hairs on your breasts are too bothersome. Any sudden increase in the hairiness of your breasts, or indeed anywhere else on your body, should send you to seek your doctor's advice.

# SIX

# Changes in the Breasts during Pregnancy

For many women, changes in their breasts are one of the first clues that they may be pregnant. The pre-menstrual tenderness, tingling and feeling of fullness will persist. This together with the missing of a period, is strongly suggestive of pregnancy. For the first few weeks of pregnancy, breasts may remain tender. The nipple area may also be super-sensitive. But after six weeks or so from the first missed period, these feelings will improve.

## Increase in size

As far as your breasts are concerned, you will still find you have an increased breast size (this is a bonus of pregnancy for small-breasted women, but unfortunately one which does not persist after pregnancy and breastfeeding are over).

This increase in size is due to an increase in both the glandular substance of the breasts and also to an increase in the amount of fat between these gland cells. Both these effects are directly due to alterations in the hormonal balance in your body. The tiny sebaceous glands on the areola, known as Montgomery's tubercles (see page 12), will also become more prominent, again due to hormonal action. You may also notice a fine network of bluish, superficial veins appearing over the surface of the breasts. It is sensible at this early stage to review your bra position. A larger cup size may well be more comfortable; also check that your bras really are providing necessary support and comfort.

### Darkening of the skin

From about the twelfth week of pregnancy on, you will notice a darkening of the skin over the nipple and areola areas of your breasts. This is more noticeable in dark-skinned women than in fair-skinned or redheaded women —in fact, in the latter little change may be seen at all. This colour change is permanent and will persist throughout life following a pregnancy. Occasionally, this darkening of the skin can spread beyond the areola immediately around the nipple, and involve much of the breast. This 'secondary areola', as it is termed, will quickly fade after delivery, unlike the persistent darkening of the areola immediately around the nipple.

### Nipple changes

Nipples become more prominent and softer during pregnancy. This is in preparation for breastfeeding. Nipples need to be malleable and of a suitable shape for the baby to be able to 'latch on' firmly. Again this change, starting early on in pregnancy, is due to the action of the hormone, progesterone, on the connective tissue in this part of the breast. (Similarly, progesterone softens all the ligaments of the body. A further facet of this action that you may notice is that you will probably need half a size larger in shoes during pregnancy. Don't worry! You are not getting permanently large feet. After the birth of your baby, your feet will return to their normal shoe size again.)

There are a few exceptions to these particular changes in the nipples. Some women have flat or inverted nipples and these may not show the changes described. Help may need to be given during pregnancy under these circumstances if breastfeeding is going to be successful (see page 50).

### Stretch marks

Occasionally stretch marks—little, red thread-like marks over the surface of the breasts—can occur early on in pregnancy, particularly if a good deal of weight is put on rapidly at this time. This is due to the breakdown of the elastic tissue immediately below the surface of the skin caused by rapid stretching (see page 50). The marks commonly seen on the abdomen later in pregnancy are due to a similar cause. These stretch marks will never entirely disappear, but they will become virtually unnoticeable over time as they turn into tiny, thin white marks.

## Colostrum secretion

From around the 20th week of pregnancy onwards, the breasts may secrete a little clear, yellowish fluid. This is known as *colostrum*, and is the forerunner of milk production. Larger amounts of colostrum are produced in the first days after the birth of the baby, and at this time it contains many valuable substances for the baby's growth and protection (see Chapter 8).

## Care of the breasts during pregnancy

*Bras*

It is wise to wear a well-fitting bra which gives good support during pregnancy. Not only will this be comfortable, but it will reduce the 'pull' of the increased weight of the breasts at this time on the underlying tissues. This in turn will reduce to a minimum any sagging of the breasts at a later date. Remember it is sensible to try on a bra at this time before buying. You may well need a larger size—perhaps both a larger overall size as well as a larger cup size. Without 'trying before buying', you could well end up with an entirely unsuitable—and uncomfortable—garment. If you buy soft bras with a minimum of fastenings, they may also be suitable for wear after the birth of your baby, when you are breastfeeding. It will very much depend on the size of your breasts, however, if this type of bra will give all the support you need at this time.

During pregnancy, some women find that it is more comfortable to wear a bra throughout the 24 hours, particularly if the breasts are large and heavy. So perhaps one of the softer bras, which give less support but are more comfortable to wear, may be a good buy for night-time wear under these circumstances.

*Looking after your nipples*
For women with normal nipples, there is no need to do anything other than usual routine hygienic care during pregnancy. Midwives of a bygone era were very keen on 'hardening' the nipples ready for breastfeeding. These procedures involved the application of surgical spirit and scrubbing of the nipple with a soft brush! Very traumatic and uncomfortable—and quite unnecessary.

Any excess secretion, particularly during the latter stages of pregnancy, will need to be gently washed away at normal bathtime. But this is all that needs to be done.

Women with flat or inverted nipples could run into difficulties with breastfeeding at a later date unless extra care is given during pregnancy. Unless nipples protrude sufficiently for the baby to take the nipple fully into his mouth, breastfeeding will prove difficult. Many previously flat or inverted nipples will alter to a more suitable shape during pregnancy due to the general softening of the tissues. But there still remain a few nipples that are persistently inverted. The wearing of a plastic nipple-shield daily, inside the bra, will often do much to improve the shape of this type of nipple. Nipple-shields are usually made of plastic, and are dome-shaped, with a hole at the apex of the dome through which the nipple should protrude. The pressure of the 'cuff' of the shield pushing on the areola of the nipple will help in pushing the nipple forward. The wearing of these shields during the day for the last few months of pregnancy, together with gentle massage around the base of the nipple and gently pulling the nipple forward, will be effective in producing a good shape in all but the most inverted of nipples.

*What to do about stretch marks*
Little can be done to entirely eliminate these tiny marks

from appearing, apart from ensuring that your overall body weight does not increase too rapidly during the early pregnancy days. Start at day one of your pregnancy, if possible, by eating sensibly and *not* starving yourself, but certainly not 'eating for two'. Adequate protein and plenty of fresh fruit and vegetables together with adequate 'roughage' foods should keep excess weight down. Small frequent meals, instead of two large ones, are preferable at this time to help avoid the nausea and sickness of early pregnancy.

Rubbing oil or cream into your breasts will, unfortunately, do little to eliminate stretch marks. It is the breaking up of the elastic tissue under the surface of the skin that is the cause of stretch marks, and no oil or cream can prevent this.

Pregnancy and subsequent breastfeeding are the prime anatomical and physiological reasons for breasts. They fulfil this task most wonderfully and efficiently, with little help other than keeping the body usually healthy.

# SEVEN

# Breastfeeding

Probably more has been written about breastfeeding over the years than any other physiological function of our bodies. The La Lèche League exists solely to promote and encourage all aspects of breastfeeding. The National Childbirth Trust also puts breastfeeding high on the list of priorities. Alongside these specialized organizations, put the help and advice that every woman receives (or should receive) on breastfeeding from midwives, doctors and health visitors, and you can see that breastfeeding is at last being given the encouragement it deserves.

## Historical aspects of breastfeeding

Until the early part of this century, breast milk was the only form of nutriment available to newborn babies. If the mother was unable to feed her own baby for some reason, a 'wet-nurse' was found who could supply the necessary breast milk for the young baby. Wet-nursing was common practice amongst the aristocracy, freeing the mother to continue her life away from the ties of frequent breast-feeding. Wet-nurses had to be women who had recently borne a child. As long as 'nursing' (or breastfeeding) continued, breast milk continued to flow with the suckling of a baby. In this way women could suckle for many months—their services were life-saving in circumstances where illness of the mother (or even death—a not uncommon occurrence) prevented breastfeeding.

But in the 1930s and 1940s, formula milks, based on cow's milk, became available in modified forms. With more women working outside the home (and this escalated during the war years when women became a vital part of the labour force) the idea of feeding their babies from a bottle became increasingly popular. Anyone who was available to care for the baby could give the feed, thus releasing the mother from always being available to feed her baby.

As the years passed, formula milks became more and more sophisticated. Breast milk and cow's milk were analysed down to the last detail. Cow's milk was modified (or 'humanized'!) until its constituents were as near to those of human milk as possible. During the 1950s and 1960s breastfeeding reached an all-time low. Fortunately, during the late 1970s and early 1980s, there has been a slow, but steady, groundswell of feeling towards the realization of the vital importance of stable mothering during a child's early life. And this also includes a resurgence in interest in breastfeeding. There are studies, both large and small, continuing throughout the country which suggest that more mothers are now breastfeeding their babies—and for a longer time—than in 1975, the year of the last national study on *Infant Feeding Practices in England and Wales* (published by HMSO in 1978). This study makes fascinating reading, and showed among many other things that, although 50 per cent of women started off breastfeeding their babies, fewer than 10 per cent of these women were still feeding their babies after two weeks—that is, by the time mother and baby had settled down together at home. This falls far short of the ideal pattern of breast milk for babies up to the age of four to six months. But looking at up-to-date figures of small studies, it would seem the pattern is now beginning to change.

## Present-day attitudes to breastfeeding

This can be looked at from two differing viewpoints—that of the breastfeeding mother herself and that of the public in general.

*Breastfeeding mothers*
There are many reasons why women choose not to breast-feed their babies, for example:

- too time-consuming
- 'tied' to the baby, and cannot take up work outside the home
- no-one else can take over feeding
- embarrassment
- worry at not being able to judge exactly how much milk the baby has taken
- has heard horrific stories from 'friends', of breastfeeding problems

All these concerns and worries are, of course, quite valid. But with help from husbands, relatives, midwives and health visitors, breastfeeding can become a source of great satisfaction to a new mother.

*The public in general*
Little help is given to accommodate the needs of breastfeeding mothers in our society today. Babies—especially in the early days—need frequent feeding, and (as will be seen later) it is vital that this is done if breastfeeding is to be successful. Babies cannot wait until their mothers reach a suitable place where feeding can take place! There is a marginal increase in the facilities in our larger city stores where breastfeeding mothers can sit quietly to feed their babies. But there is still a long way to go before mothers can feel certain of finding a suitable place to feed their babies.

There is also still much embarrassment at women feeding their babies in public. Even if the breastfeeding mother is happy to do this, she can be easily put off by the reaction of the people around her.

Ideally, there should be adequate facilities at all major airports, railway and bus stations, shops etc., where mothers can comfortably—and warmly—feed and change their babies. Recent progress has been made in this direction. A new national baby care symbol will soon be appearing in public places showing that facilities are available for parents with babies and young children. This symbol will indicate that certain minimum criteria have been met in the way of warmth, cleanliness, privacy, etc. A number of organizations have been involved with this progressive step, and they will be monitoring places showing the symbol in order that standards are maintained.

## Benefits of breastfeeding

There is no doubt whatsoever of the benefits of breast milk to babies. Even a very short period of breastfeeding—two to three weeks—can be of great benefit to a baby. The milk is readily available at exactly the right temperature and of exactly the right constituency for each individual baby whenever it is needed. Add to this the warm snug security of your mother's arms and the familiar smell of her body and it is no wonder that successfully breastfed babies are content. But in a book about the breast, what are the benefits to the mother of breastfeeding her baby?

1 High on the list comes the increasing ability to 'bond' with your baby if you are breastfeeding. The close

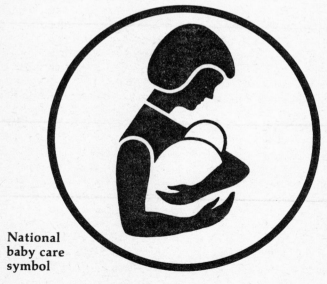

National
baby care
symbol

relationship involved in breastfeeding creates an easy atmosphere in which you can fall in love with your baby (by no means the spontaneous surge of rapture at birth so beloved of magazine stories). Of course bottle-feeding mothers will also develop this 'bonding' with their babies, but breastfeeding makes this so much easier.

2 Breastfeeding stimulates contractions of the uterus (see 'after-pains', page 58). Over the first six weeks of baby's life, this will assist in the return of the uterus to its normal size. This in turn will help with the return of the figure to normal.

3 Preceding this return of the uterus to normal within six weeks, putting the baby to the breast immediately after birth will assist in the delivery of the placenta—or 'afterbirth'. This tissue, which has nourished the baby throughout the nine months of pregnancy, is expelled within around 20 minutes of the baby's birth. Putting the baby to the breast releases hormones which cause contractions of the uterus. So there is less likelihood of problems of complete delivery of the placenta with immediate breastfeeding.

4 It is still controversial whether or not breastfeeding protects women against subsequent breast cancer. Previous studies in Japan pointed towards a protective effect of breastfeeding. But Japan has a low incidence of breast cancer anyway, and there may be other factors at work producing these low figures of the disease. The classical study amongst the boat women of Hong Kong who only fed from the right breast showed a lower incidence of cancer in this breast, as compared with the left breast. In women from the same area in whom the right-breasted feeding did not apply, breast cancers were equal in both breasts. But other studies have not proved this theory. On the other side of the coin, no study has ever suggested that breastfeeding leads to an increased incidence of cancer.

## How breastfeeding works

The production of milk in the breasts is a highly complex

process. Milk is produced by the milk glands in the breast tissue. The necessary nutrients and fluids to produce this milk are obtained ultimately from the blood supply to these glands. The whole process is under the control of a number of hormones (chemical 'messengers') produced in various parts of the body: the pituitary, thyroid and adrenal glands. A particular hormone called prolactin is the main hormone concerned. It is produced by the pituitary gland, deep in the brain. At around the tenth week of pregnancy this hormone can be measured in the blood. The level of prolactin gradually increases throughout pregnancy, so that at the time of the birth of the baby it is at its highest level. It is responsible for the production of the small amount of colostrum during the latter weeks of pregnancy. Acting together with prolactin, but in a negative way, is the hormone oestrogen from the placenta. The high levels of oestrogen from this source throughout pregnancy ensure that full milk production is not initiated during pregnancy. At the birth of the baby, these oestrogen levels fall, the inhibiting effects of this hormone cease, so prolactin can act fully and start full milk production. But this is not the full story! Prolactin secretion is further stimulated by the actual sucking of the baby on the nipple. So to fully 'turn on the system' it is necessary that the baby be put to the breast at frequent intervals.

Between feeds milk is continually being produced in the milk-producing glands in the breast. Some of this is stored in the reservoirs immediately behind the areola of the nipple. This is known as the 'fore-milk', and ensures that the baby obtains milk as soon as he begins to suck. The 'hind-milk', will pass into the milk ducts by the action of tiny muscles in the breast tissue as the baby sucks. The process when this milk passes into the milk ducts is known as the 'letdown' reflex. It will only satisfactorily occur if mother and baby are content, quiet and happy in the intimate pleasures of breastfeeding. Other factors, such as the satisfactory positioning of the baby's mouth around the areola of the nipple, are also important in the initiation of the 'letdown' reflex. It is only when the hind-milk flows into the baby's mouth that he will be satisfied. This milk contains a higher proportion of calories—mainly in the form of fat—than the fore-milk, and so forms a vital part of his nutrition.

### Establishing breastfeeding

You can see how many factors need to work together for satisfactory breastfeeding. But do remember that mothers have been breastfeeding their babies quite happily and successfully for thousands of years without having any knowledge at all of the actual mechanics of breastfeeding. All that is needed is the willingness to give your baby this wonderfully beneficial start to his life, and a little help from a sympathetic and knowledgeable midwife, health visitor, breastfeeding counsellor or friend.

Ideally babies should be put to the breast as soon after birth as possible. Babies of even a few minutes old will automatically know the function of the breast and will nuzzle and lick the nipple. This is the beginning of the chain of messages through the mother's hormonal system that milk production is now the order of the day. Over the next few hours, after both mother and baby have rested from the hard work of labour, the baby should be put to the breast frequently. As the nipple touches his cheek he will automatically turn his head and take the nipple into his mouth. This is known as the 'rooting reflex', and is one of the inbuilt mechanisms for survival. For the first few days of breastfeeding, mothers may feel a cramp-like pain in their lower stomach. This is known as 'after-pains', and is the uterus contracting down. Breastfeeding does much to help the uterus return to normal.

It is important at this early stage that the baby should be 'latched on' to the breast satisfactorily. He should not be allowed to chew on the surface of the nipple. This will only serve to make it sore—and maybe put the mother off breastfeeding for good. The whole nipple and areola should be inside the baby's mouth. His lips, forming a seal around the areola, will thus press on the reservoirs of milk immediately under the areola, and so initiate the flow of milk.

These early days of breastfeeding are when mothers will need encouragement to persevere. It is vital that they should feel comfortable and free from worry. Anxieties about other children, husbands and household cares, along with embarrassment, can so easily inhibit the 'letdown' reflex. And without this reflex acting in full measure breastfeeding will be fraught with difficulties—if not quite impossible.

## Frequency of feeds

Breastfeeding will only be successful as long as there is an adequate supply of milk. And this, as we have seen, is dependent on a number of factors which all finally hinge on the stimulation of the nipple by the baby. So, during the first few weeks of breastfeeding, demand feeding—in other words, allowing the baby to suck whenever he is restless or crying—is a vital part of the successful establishment of breastfeeding. Primitive people suckle their babies almost continually during the early days after birth, and so practically all babies are—of necessity—successfully breast-fed. As well as producing a good milk supply, this frequent suckling will have a soothing, comforting effect on the baby, so that he will cry less often.

Within a few weeks, the frequency of feeds will reduce, and usually mother and baby will settle down into an approximately four-hourly routine of feeding. But if this rigid schedule is enforced from the early days, it is doubtful if breastfeeding will be successful.

## How breast milk is made up

One of the most frequent worries voiced by breastfeeding mothers is that their milk looks thin and watery. They are naturally concerned that this milk is not of the right type to feed their baby satisfactorily. This, in fact, is far from the case. Breast milk is wonderfully adapted to meet all the needs of the growing baby however it may look. And this adaptation is also in evidence later, as the appearance of the milk alters throughout the day.

*First days after birth*
In the first day or two after birth, the breasts secrete the thin, yellowish fluid, known as colostrum, which was noticeable in small amounts during the latter weeks of pregnancy. Colostrum contains very little fat and carbo-hydrate—hence its thin, watery appearance. But it is rich in protein, minerals and vitamins, together with substances which protect the vulnerable newborn baby from infection. So you can see how important it is that the tiny baby should benefit from this if at all possible. Also, as we have seen, sucking at the breast is the very best way of stimulating the production of further milk supplies.

*Beginning of full milk production*
On the second or third day after birth full milk production will begin—or the milk will 'come in'. (Sometimes this happens with a great rush. Under these conditions it is important that the mother new to breastfeeding is given sympathetic help.) This milk will at first be bluish and watery . But as the baby sucks at the breast, stimulating the 'letdown' reflex, the milk will become thicker and more creamy-looking —in fact, very much more as most mothers expect it to look.

*Milk after breastfeeding is established*
As breastfeeding becomes established, mothers will notice that at the beginning of a feed the milk is often thinner and bluish in colour. As feeding continues the milk will become thicker and creamier; this is because it contains a higher proportion of fat that is secreted by the milk-glands being 'let down'. Perhaps one of the commonest causes of failure to breastfeed happily is that mothers are not encouraged to put their babies to the breast at frequent enough intervals. If this is the case only the thinner fore-milk is secreted, and mothers become concerned that this thin-looking milk is

not adequate for the needs of their baby. The baby will then become restless for two reasons. First, he is hungry, as the milk containing fat and carbohydrate is not reaching him. Second, he needs to suck at the breast more frequently, for comfort as well as nutrition. Mothers will then feel the need to give a formula milk by bottle and so breastfeeding becomes more infrequent. And it is then that breastfeeding begins to fail.

In a successfully breastfeeding mother, it can also be noticed that the milk changes in character throughout the day. This is dependent on many factors, one of which is the type of foods that the mother has recently been eating. There is no need to restrict yourself in any way from the eating point of view when you are breastfeeding. Beware though of 'eating for two', and putting on too much weight! You *will* need extra calories daily to breastfeed successfully without feeling tired yourself. But do not go 'overboard' about this, and eat all the fattening cakes, chocolates etc. in sight. A good varied diet with plenty of fresh fruit and vegetables, and adequate cereal roughage, should be your aim, both to supply your baby's needs and to keep yourself healthy. Certain foods, such as for example strawberries, plums or gooseberries when fresh in season, may have an effect on your baby—perhaps giving him loose motions and maybe a colicky stomach-ache. (This may happen to you also, of course, under these conditions!) This can only be discovered by trial and error. If a certain food seems to be upsetting your baby, avoid this in the future. Remember, your milk is made from the substances which you take into your own body.

This also applies to any drugs you may be taking. As far as possible, *all drugs should be avoided* by breastfeeding mothers unless absolutely necessary for their own health or a particular condition. Any necessary long-term drug regime must be monitored carefully by your doctor. Obviously, the odd aspirin for a headache will create few problems, but if you find you are needing these at regular intervals, your doctor should be contacted. It is as well to stop smoking altogether and to reduce alcohol intake to a minimum while breastfeeding. These rules also apply, of course, during pregnancy.

## Bras during breastfeeding

Most women will feel more comfortable in a bra while they are breastfeeding. There is no good medical reason for wearing a bra when breastfeeding—or at any other time. But during lactation, the breasts are full and heavy and a well-fitting bra will often feel more comfortable.

There are special 'nursing' bras available. These have a front flap and fastening that can easily be undone at feed-times. But many women find that it is just as easy to pull down—or up—an ordinary bra at feed-times. Obviously the size must be correct, and will probably be larger than the size you usually buy. So be sure that you get the size that is comfortable and does not cut into your breasts. You may well find that you need to buy three bras. Milk can leak from your breasts between feeds and stain the bra, so that frequent washing is necessary.

## Possible problems

*Engorgement*
Engorgement of the breasts can frequently occur in the second or third day after the birth of the baby when the full milk supply comes in. The breasts become tense, swollen and exquisitely tender. Even the 'tail' of the breast up into the armpit becomes involved and is similarly painful. Some women can also feel hot and shivery and run a fever at this time. All these symptoms are due to the sudden inrush of milk from the milk glands blocking the blood and lymph vessels. Due to this pressure, fluid leaks out into the connective framework of the breast tissue, and so adds to the general swelling and discomfort.

The way to treat—and avoid—engorgement of the breasts is to feed your baby frequently. Have him beside your bed, and as soon as you are aware that he is restless put him to the breast. The alternative is to express some milk, either by hand or with the help of a breast-pump. If your baby is initially a reluctant or a sleepy feeder, this latter course of action may be necessary for a few days. Sometimes the engorgement is so excessive that the nipple appears buried in the surrounding swollen breast tissue. Under these circumstances a nipple-shield may be helpful in enabling your baby to suck satisfactorily. Flannels wrung out in cold water can also help ease the heat and tenderness of the engorged breast, and aspirin may be necessary to relieve the pain. It is obviously better to avoid engorgement altogether by frequent breastfeeding. But if it does occur, this particular problem can be overcome with sympathetic help and understanding.

*Cracked nipples*
This is probably one of the most common reasons why breastfeeding is abandoned. A crack in the delicate tissue of the nipple is extremely painful, and the last thing a mother with a cracked nipple feels like doing is feeding her baby. But if the milk supply is to be kept up this is just what must be done, or alternatively, milk must be expressed at regular intervals.

But what is the cause of a cracked nipple? Several factors can be involved in this painful condition:

1 Poor 'positioning' of the baby on the nipple in the early days of breastfeeding can lead to a cracked nipple. If the areola of the breast is not taken into the baby's mouth, but he is allowed to chew on the nipple instead, conditions are ripe for this condition. Similarly, if the baby sucks at the nipple in a lopsided manner (possibly of necessity due to the position in which he is held) this can put excessive pull on one part of the nipple. So help in the earliest days of feeding is of vital importance to the mother in order to avoid this particular problem.
2 Nipples can become wet and soggy when encased in a bra for many hours every day. If breast milk leaks out between feeds this problem is compounded. Thus the delicate surface of the nipple can be easily broken when

the baby starts to suck. To avoid this, a cotton bra is preferable to one made of a synthetic material. The cotton is more absorbent as well as letting a modicum of air through to the nipple. Also, if at all possible, allow your nipple to be exposed to the air for some part of the day. Leaving some breast milk to dry on the surface of the nipple before putting on a bra again can also be helpful in forming a protective coat for the nipple.

3 It is a fact that women who breastfeed their babies frequently have fewer problems with cracked and sore nipples.

To treat a cracked nipple, which possibly is constantly being reopened in spite of all your preventive measures, you may have to stop feeding from this one breast for 24 to 48 hours. It is vital, however, if you wish to continue breastfeeding, that you express the milk from this breast. This will ensure that the milk supply is kept going until your baby can again stimulate production.

If the crack has been inflamed or infected by thrush (a fungus), your doctor will need to prescribe special antibiotic cream to clear up the problem.

### Blocked ducts and mastitis
This condition is basically a localized engorgement. One section of the milk duct system becomes blocked due to:

1 Again, improper positioning of the baby on the breast.
2 Pressure from an ill-fitting or tight bra.
3 Insufficient emptying of the breast by infrequent feeds.

### Symptoms

1 A tender, lumpy swelling over one part of the breast.
2 A hot and shivering feeling as with generalized engorgement.

*Treatment*

1 Be sure that your baby is sucking properly and firmly on to the areola, and that you are not wearing any tight clothing over your breasts.

2 Massage your breast gently towards the nipple over the tender lumpy portion.

3 A covered hot water bottle can sometimes help the flow of milk.

4 If this treatment does not help in 24 hours, or if your breast becomes hot and shiny over the lump, contact your doctor. It is possible that infection has occurred in the stagnating milk in the blocked duct, causing mastitis. A course of antibiotics will be necessary along with the routine treatment for a blocked duct. There is no need to stop feeding your baby under these conditions. In fact regular frequent feeding will help.

*Breast abscess*

This occurs following on from an inadequately treated mastitis. The infection becomes localized in one part of the breast, and an extremely painful, red swelling develops with pus formation. Medical treatment is necessary for this condition. A prolonged course of antibiotics may clear the infection, but surgical drainage of the abscess may be necessary.

## Reasons why breastfeeding fails

*Insufficient help*

Insufficient help given to inexperienced mothers in the early days of breastfeeding is probably the commonest cause of failure. Breastfeeding is an art that has to be learned these days. Bygone generations, and primitive peoples, intuitively knew how to 'nurse' their babies, and much support was given in the early days to a breastfeeding mother. Regrettably today, this intuitive art has largely been lost. But signs are that women are beginning once again to take an interest in, and to 'develop a feel' for, breastfeeding their babies.

*Domestic problems*

On returning home from hospital, many mothers find household cares and the needs of other children and family members make breastfeeding come a poor second to these other activities. She is tired after the hard work of pregnancy and labour, time is at a premium, and she is unable to relax sufficiently to allow her body to produce the milk in adequate quantities for her baby's needs. The necessary time for 'demand' feeding is just not available. So the milk supply diminishes, the baby is hungry and cries, and bottle-feeding is introduced. And until we realize that mothers need time to get to know their babies and to feed them with a minimum of everyday cares for a while, this state of affairs will continue. Much help can be given by relatives and friends taking over routine chores for a week or two. Mothers can also help themselves by allowing their standards to drop temporarily. A layer of dust will harm no-one, but a week or two spent in establishing breastfeeding will be of inestimable value to a new baby.

*'Difficult feeders'*

Some babies are initially reluctant to breastfeed. This may be because:

1 They are sleepy following excess drugs necessary in labour.
2 The baby is tired from crying—this can occur if feed-times are scheduled and at regular intervals, and the baby is allowed to become hungry and lonely.
3 Breasts are engorged and it is difficult to get an adequate grip on the nipple.
4 Nipples are inverted or flat—here again the baby will have difficulty in finding the nipple.

Most, if not all, of these problems can be resolved by sympathetic and knowledgeable help in the early days of breastfeeding.

*Unwillingness or embarrassment in mothers*

Many women are reluctant to breastfeed early in pregnancy, largely due to ignorance of what is actually involved, and how breastfeeding works. With good antenatal tuition, and full explanations of the benefits of breastfeeding, as well as detailed instruction on how to breastfeed successfully, many mothers will change their minds, and by the time their baby is born will be keen to breastfeed.

## Difficult conditions for breastfeeding

Finally, there are a few special conditions in which breastfeeding may be particularly difficult.

*Premature babies* whose sucking reflex is immature may have difficulties. Here skilled help is necessary and maybe expressed breast milk may be the answer for a while.

*Babies with deformities* around the mouth—for example, harelip and cleft palate—will find 'latching on' to the breast difficult or even impossible. Here again expressed breast milk will have to be given by special bottle or spoon together with later surgical procedures.

*Twins* can present special problems in timing and positioning of feeds. But many mothers successfully breastfeed their twins. Once a routine is established, together with help for the mother, breastfeeding twins can be as easy as feeding just one baby.

*Illness in the mother* can of course preclude breastfeeding altogether. But this is dependent on the type of illness. Medical advice, taking into account the needs of both mother and baby, is necessary under these conditions.

Breastfeeding is the main physiological function of the breasts. Much care and help needs to be given these days to encourage women to use their breasts for this purpose. Fears of spoiling the silhouette of their figures are largely unfounded, and the advantage to the baby of breastfeeding is immeasurable. Breast care needs a little more time and expertise during pregnancy and lactation, but the benefits are well worth this extra effort.

*Part 3*
*The Mature Breast*

# EIGHT

# Breast Care after 40

The age at which breast changes are noticeable in maturity is, of course, quite arbitrary and varies markedly from woman to woman. Along with all other aspects of physical characteristics, we are all quite unique. And, along with other facets of ageing, breast changes occur only slowly over a number of years, and so gradually that any difference in silhouette is imperceptible to a woman looking at her figure day after day. It is only when she compares her present-day figure with a photograph of—say —20 years earlier, that the changes in her bust-line are obvious.

There are several changes that account for these differences. In the years between approximately 40 to 60, the glandular tissue in the breast diminishes. It is usually no longer necessary for the breasts to fulfil the function for which they were intended, namely breastfeeding babies. So the active part of the breast tissue—the milk glands and associated structures—become smaller through disuse. If a late baby arrives, however, this tissue will again become active and breastfeeding will be possible, as before. It has been known for grandmothers to be able to breastfeed their grandchildren when—under extreme conditions of deprivation—this has been necessary. And also women adopting children have been able to breastfeed if sufficient stimulation, by frequent suckling, has been given—yet one more facet of the amazing adaptability of the human body under differing circumstances.

Alongside this diminution in glandular tissue goes an increase in the fibrous tissue content of the breast. In addition to this increase, women of around 40 to 50 years of age do tend to put on weight! This means that there is also an increase in the fat content of the tissues of the breast as

71

well as elsewhere in the body. So overall, the addition of extra fat and fibrous tissue compensates for the diminution in glandular tissue. This means, in fact, that there is probably little change during these years in the shape and size of the breasts. Many women notice at this time of life that their nipples become excessively sensitive, and occasionally the nipple area becomes red and swollen. Check that your bra is not rubbing this delicate tissue. Perhaps a change to a soft, seamless bra could provide the solution. If this persists for too long, or the nipple is very red and swollen, a visit to your doctor is advisable.

All these changes are due to the differing levels of hormones being secreted at this time of life—the menopause or 'change of life'. This 'change' occurs at different times in different women, some women starting in the early 40s and other women beginning the process ten years later. The most obvious sign of the onset of the menopause is, of course, the irregularity—and finally cessation—of the regular monthly period. But other wide-reaching changes also occur in many other organs and systems of the body. And breasts are no exception to this.

Later on in life, in the late 50s and early 60s, most women will notice that their breasts begin to sag and become less firm, due to a diminution in the fat content of the breast (obviously in overweight women this facet will not be noticeable). Along with this cause for drooping breasts is a general weakening of connective tissue all over the body. The connective tissue framework of the breast is not exempt from this laxity, so breasts tend to sag to a greater extent.

This may sound like a gloomy picture for the mature woman for whom, after all, life has certainly not finished. But do remember that all these changes are so imperceptible that you will probably be quite unaware of them for many years. There is good reason for avoiding any drastic slimming regimes in the middle years if you want your bust silhouette to remain youthful for as long as possible.

Check your bra at this time. Possibly a smaller cup size

and different style may suit you better than the one you have been accustomed to buying for many years.

## Care of breasts

This should continue as throughout the rest of life—no special treatment other than washing as with the rest of the body. If the breasts are heavy and pendulous, remember to dry thoroughly underneath to avoid skin rashes occurring in this situation. Skin can get very moist, red and sore unless particular care is taken.

*Self-examination*

The one facet of care that you must be sure to continue during the mature years is the routine self-examination of the breasts. The incidence of cancer of the breast (along with all other cancers elsewhere in the body) is higher in women over 40 years of age. So it is vitally important that you continue the habit that you have, hopefully, acquired earlier in life of examining each part of each breast once every month. In this way you will find the smallest lump. And remember, early diagnosis means that treatment can be given early should a cancerous lump be found. This will offer the very best chance of cure. You will have to set yourself a new routine once your periods have ceased. Whereas you were able, by your periods, to remember the recurring dates when you should examine your breast, this will no longer be available to you. So why not tick off—for example—on your kitchen calendar the date when you last did your routine breast examination? Perhaps the first day of each month is a good idea. The procedure is exactly the same as when you were younger (see page 30). For extra information and details on self-examination of breasts there are two excellent leaflets available:

- *Breast Self-examination*, from
  The Health Education Council
  78 New Oxford Street
  London WC1

● *Everyone's Doing the Breast-Test*, from
Women's National Cancer Control Campaign
1 South Audley Street
London W1Y 5DQ

Women's attitudes to examining their breasts are very variable.

1 Among older women who have not been brought up with today's young women's knowledge of various screening procedures for certain conditions (for example, the smear test for cancer of the cervix, routine blood pressure measurement for raised blood pressure, etc.) there is often a reluctance to examine their own bodies. This is a difficult 'hang-up' to overcome, but one which you should try to beat, as the benefits of screening procedures— and certainly breast self-examination—are proven.

2 It is not uncommon to hear women of all ages state that the reason why they do not examine their breasts regularly is that they 'do not want to know' if they have any lump in their breast. Again, a difficult attitude to counter, but why not try discussing this with several other women? Their views will probably be different from yours and they may well convince you of your erroneous thinking.

3 Many women also give 'lip-service' to breast self-examination. They will do the test in a rushed, half-hearted, superficial way and then breathe a sigh of relief that all appears to be normal. In reality, they could be fooling themselves. Unless the test is done *systematically* and *thoroughly*, the smallest lump can be easily missed— and remember, it is the *smallest* lump that you are trying to find.

4 It is easy to forget that there are conditions of the breast, other than cancer, that can be found by regular self-examination. And these conditions can frequently be easily and wholly successfully treated. Hand in hand with this attitude goes uncertainty of what to look for in the breast other than the ubiquitous 'lump'. So, try to find a

clinic specializing in women's conditions locally, or a series of talks about the subject, and go along to learn.

Concern is felt by members of the health professions about these various facets of (understandable) attitudes to self-examination of breasts in women. There is no doubt that routine performance of this simple test can be instrumental in preventing a good deal of the misery of advanced breast disease—and this includes conditions of the breast other than cancer. Various surveys have been carried out on the best ways to encourage women to examine their breasts adequately in a routine way. The most successful ways of encouragement would seem to be threefold:

1 Meetings held amongst women in a wide range of settings—for example, housewives' groups, Women's Institutes, well-women clinics, etc.—where information can be given by knowledgeable staff. The normal anatomy and physiology of the breast can be discussed and taught here as well as discussions on the various signs and symptoms of any potential problems. Specialized leaflets, such as those mentioned on pages 73–4 can then be distributed to act as an *'aide-mémoire'* to the women when they subsequently perform the breast test at home. Films and tapes should be available for use in such circumstances.
2 Demonstration of the technique of breast self-examination on a one-to-one basis in the clinic situation is an ideal way of giving and gaining confidence.
3 Following on from the demonstration can be the *practice under supervision* by women themselves. They will then feel more secure in the knowledge: (a) of exactly what they are looking for; and (b) that they are doing the job properly.

In a few parts of the country this ideal is practised, but is very much dependent on local facilities and enthusiasm.

## Other methods of detecting and diagnosing breast conditions

Besides the all-important monthly self-examination of the breast that all women should be encouraged to perform themselves, there are other 'screening' procedures that can be done to detect disease. A screening procedure is one which aims to discover a disease process before the sufferer has any symptoms. In this way, the disease (whatever it may be) can be treated at the earliest possible moment, thus giving greater chances of cure. Other, widely differing, examples of screening procedures are the cervical smear test for cancer of the cervix, and the 'heel prick' (or Guthrie) test on newborn babies for the disease known as phenyl-ketonuria.

In some parts of the country *Well-Women Clinics* are run. These take very many different forms, ranging from clinics which perform a number of tests at one visit—for example, a cervical smear test, an examination of the breasts, along with other specific tests for anaemia, raised blood pressure, urinary infection and diabetes, etc. Other specialized clinics, such as family planning clinics, will also 'screen' women for breast disease in addition to giving contraceptive advice. These clinics also usually provide literature on the method and importance of self-examination of the breasts.

In addition to the basic clinical test of feeling the breasts systematically to discover any unusual thickening or swelling, there are a number of specialized tests that can be carried out.

*Mammography*
This is a procedure which involves X-ray examination of the breast. With good, sensitive apparatus and skilled operators and interpreters of the X-ray picture, very small swellings in the breast can be seen. It is important that this procedure (and indeed all other specialized procedures in this field) should be preceded by clinical examination of the breast.

This test is a very specialized one, and results must be correlated with the results of other checks. It is not advisable to submit women—and particularly young women —to unnecessary X-ray examinations, although with today's sophisticated X-ray machines, the 'dose' of X-rays given in any one examination is minimal. Also, the interpretation of the results is more difficult in younger women, where the breast tissue is denser than that of older women.

For all these reasons mammography is not used routinely as a screening procedure for breast disease. But it is a valuable procedure under certain specific conditions:

1 To help to determine if there are any swellings in a large breast which is difficult to examine adequately.
2 To help to sort out the cause of a lump or thickening that has been felt in the breast; under this heading can also be included the additional help this particular form of X-ray examination can give to other breast symptoms such as discharge from the nipple or breast pain.
3 If a lump has been found in one breast, the other breast can usefully be examined by X-ray as it is important to be sure that breast disease is not also affecting the other breast.

Many women are concerned that X-ray examination (particularly of something as delicate as breast tissue) may actually cause cancer. These fears are unnecessary for two reasons:

1 X-ray machines today deliver only the smallest possible amount of radiation in any one X-ray film. This is in direct contrast to the X-ray machines of the early days when considerable radiation was spread around the whole vicinity of the examination.
2 Mammography is not undertaken lightly or indiscriminately. Much care, thought and research has gone—and is still going on—into the best ways of detecting breast disease by this means.

*Thermography*
This method of screening relies on the fact that some

cancers of the breast emit heat. This small temperature change (about 1°C) can be measured by specialized techniques.

Thermography is a relatively easy and harmless method of detecting breast disease. No X-rays are used and the breast is not handled at all. Perhaps the only rather tedious part of the examination is the ten minutes or so in which women have to sit in a uniformly heated room with bare breasts. This is necessary in order to be sure that the breast tissue is at the same temperature as the surrounding atmosphere. The actual 'test' only takes a few minutes.

Unfortunately, thermography is not 100 per cent reliable, for several reasons:

1 Only around two-thirds of breast cancers emit heat; so a potentially serious condition can be missed if this test alone is done.
2 Other conditions of the breast—an infected spot, sunburn or an underlying chest infection can also give rise to 'hot spots' being shown. So unless especial care is taken to eliminate these kinds of causes of a raised breast temperature, false results can be obtained.

But thermography can usefully be used in addition to other methods of detecting disease—as long as the necessary apparatus is available, of course.

*Ultrasound*
Ultrasound is the passage of high-frequency sound waves through a specific part of the body. This examination is widely used in pregnancy, as many women will know, to determine accurately the size and position of the baby. These waves bounce back from organs or swellings of differing densities and are visualized on a television screen. Much skill is needed to interpret the results of the pictures thus gained and, unfortunately, the smaller lumps cannot be detected by this form of investigation. So the very early stages of disease, which all tests are trying to discover, are the very ones that can be missed by an ultrasonic scan.

These then are the methods of screening for breast disease, and primarily cancer, in women. All methods have their limitations in one form or another. But the very best way of detecting the smallest lump is by *all* women examining their own breasts *properly* on a *regular* basis. As we have seen this can also have its problems, but with a little knowledge, discussion and gaining of expertise much of this can be overcome.

In both Britain and Europe there are ongoing trials into the best ways of screening women for breast cancer using one, or a combination, of all the various techniques available. Results from these trials, in a few years time, will give much useful information and set guidelines for future methods of screening.

# NINE

# Problems in the Mature Breast

Talk about disease of the breast in women over 40 years of age, and everyone will immediately think that the only condition of which you are talking is cancer. But while cancer does, of course, occur more commonly in this age group, it is by no means the only condition that affects the mature breast. Other conditions include fibrocystic disease, benign (non-cancerous) lumps, duct ectasia and certain other conditions outside the breast tissue, but which can give rise to pain associated with the breast.

## Fibrocystic disease

This condition (see also pages 24 and 42), as well as occurring in young women, also affects older women, especially around the time of the menopause. As in the adolescent girl, the hormonal changes at this time of life have much to do with the incidence of the disease. You will become aware of a problem by either discomfort in the affected breast, or by the discovery of a swelling during your routine breast check.

An early appointment with the doctor must be the first course of action if a discovery of this kind is made. He will refer you to a doctor specializing in breast disease. If cystic formation is part of the disease process, the specialist will probably need to remove some of the fluid content of the cyst. This is done both from a curative and a diagnostic point of view. The fluid withdrawn will be put on a slide and looked at under a microscope. This is a valuable diagnostic procedure, as the picture of the cells will show if there are any malignant (or cancerous) cells. If this *is* the case, further investigation must be done (see Chapter 10). A cancerous lump can co-exist with fibrocystic disease. But if no malignant cells are seen under the microscope, there is no remaining lump after the aspiration—and the cyst does not refill with fluid after one or two aspirations—this relatively simple procedure can be a curative one. (Obviously this technique when used as a diagnostic procedure must be accompanied by the results from other forms of breast examination.)

## Benign lumps

### Intra-duct papilloma
This is a small, wart-like growth which occurs in one or other of the ducts of the breast just under the nipple. It can occur at any age, but is probably more common in the older woman (see page 41). The commonest early symptom is a discharge from the nipple, but occasionally it is only a small, hard pea-like swelling under the nipple area that will point to an intra-duct papilloma.

Surgical treatment, under a general anaesthetic, is necessary to remove this growth. These papillomata can recur and can become cancerous, so regular check-ups are necessary for several years after surgery for this condition.

### Duct ectasia
This is a somewhat similar condition affecting the milk ducts immediately beneath the nipple, where a small lump may be felt. A sticky discharge is also a common symptom and frequently both breasts are affected. Surgical treatment can be necessary. Duct ectasia most commonly occurs in women over 40 years of age, but it is not a cancerous condition.

### Lipoma
This is a fatty tissue lump and has a very specific 'feel'. Again, specialized advice must be sought. In this older age group it is probable that the surgeon will want to remove this type of swelling to be quite sure that there are no associated cancerous changes.

Along somewhat similar lines is a condition known as *fat*

*necrosis.* Associated with ageing goes the process by which fatty tissue is replaced by tough fibrous tissue. This can give rise to an irregularly shaped hard lump in the breast. As this can feel very similar to a cancerous lump it is necessary to have it removed surgically. Diagnosis can be helped under these conditions by mammography (see page 00), as the calcium that this type of swelling sometimes contains is clearly visible on this form of test.

*Fibrosis*
Fibrosis of the breast tissue is a common occurrence in the breasts of older women. There are two common areas where this occurs:

1 The part of the breast where the breast is attached to the chest wall is probably the most usual place (possibly the continual rubbing of a bra has some bearing on this).
2 The top upper quarter of the breast.

If you feel this type of thickening—as opposed to a well-rounded lump—you should seek your doctor's advice. Chances are high that this is merely yet another aspect of ageing. But it is wise to check thoroughly that this is not an early manifestation of a cancerous lump.

## Other conditions

There are a few other conditions affecting structures near to the breast which can give rise to concern that the symptoms are arising in the breast itself. In the older woman there are three main conditions that can be mistaken for breast disease unless the true cause is diagnosed; all these have pain in the breast area as their main symptom: angina, chondritis, and shingles.

*Angina*
This is the condition caused by heart disease which gives pain in the chest, especially on any extra physical effort. In some women this pain can seem to arise in their breast.

Your doctor will be able to sort out the true cause by hearing what you have to tell him about the type, timing and distribution of your pain and by examining your heart and lungs as well as your breast. Treatment must be of the underlying condition.

*Chondritis*

This is a low-grade inflammatory condition of the cartilage which attaches the ribs to the breastbone. A physical strain—perhaps through over-violent gardening or other form of exercise—can often initiate this condition, which can be painful. The pain is often felt in one or other of the breasts. Treatment is rest and avoidance of further strain on this part of the body, and analgesics to control the pain.

*Shingles*

This is a viral infection (closely akin to chickenpox) which can affect nerve-endings over part of the breast. It is associated with a typical rash but, before this rash appears, there can be severe pain over the area affected by the infection. As soon as the rash appears the diagnosis is clear.

# TEN

# Cancer of the Breast

This is a condition about which every woman has heard, and is the one diagnosis dreaded by any woman finding a lump in her breast. So a few statistics will perhaps put this condition into perspective.

1 Around 80 per cent of all breast lumps are found to be due to causes other than cancer.
2 Only around 8 per cent of all women will suffer from breast cancer.
3 The majority of breast cancers occur in older women. These cancers are slow growing in about 50 per cent. So with early treatment the chances of many trouble-free years are high.

But on the negative side, it must be remembered that:

1 Around 30 per cent of all cancers in women are cancers of the breast.
2 About 15,000 women will die as a result of breast cancer in Britain every year.

But remember two further facts:

1 Many of these women will be well advanced in years.
2 Double this number will die from other infections such as pneumonia, etc.

Figures and statistics are all very well! It is when *you* actually have the disease that your mind is focused on its possible causes. Also, what should be your course of action if you discover a lump in your breast? And, perhaps most important of all, what will be the treatment possible for this worrying condition?

# Factors which may influence the possibility of a breast cancer

Unfortunately there is no one cause which can be incriminated in the development of a breast cancer in a particular woman. (This is also true of all other cancers.) But there are several interesting facts which have come to light over the years by various research projects, and by looking at the numbers of women suffering from breast cancer on a worldwide basis. Obviously all these factors will not apply to any one woman, and indeed it is virtually impossible to say with certainty what was the cause of one woman's cancer. But it is interesting to be aware of the possibilities that are considered to have a bearing on incidence of the disease.

*Genetic factors*

If a close relative has suffered from a cancer of the breast, the chances are higher that other female members of the family will also suffer from the disease. This fact, if this applies in your family, makes it even more important that you must examine your breasts carefully every month. Also advisable is regular attendance at a well-woman clinic, or other clinic that is available locally, for checking out your findings on your own monthly examination. And, of course, it is very important that you should contact your doctor as soon as possible if you find anything unusual in your breast.

*Breastfeeding*

There has been much controversy over the years as to whether women who breastfeed their babies are less likely to develop breast cancer than their sisters who bottle-feed. Research reports from all over the world have been at variance. The theory behind the protective effects of breastfeeding is the high prolactin (a hormone produced during breastfeeding, see page 57) produced during this activity. But some authorities think that unless 'demand' feeding of a high frequency is undertaken, the hormonal levels reached are insignificant.

But one positive fact emerges: in no way does breastfeeding have any *deleterious* effect on the mother, either at the time of breastfeeding or later in her life.

### Childbearing

Having a baby early in life—within the first ten years after starting menstruating—does seem to afford protection against a later cancer of the breast. The earlier in reproductive life is the pregnancy the better protection would seem to be given. Childless women run a higher risk of breast cancer than do women who have children. But oddly, women who have their first babies over the age of 35 years have an even higher incidence of breast cancer than childless women. So it would seem that the changes in the hormonal levels arising during pregnancy are important in the development of cancerous cells in the breast.

### Diet

This may seem a remote subject to discuss in the context of breast cancer! Cancer of the digestive system—yes—but the breast would seem to be far removed from any possible effects. It is all back to the hormone picture again. For example, a diet high in fat (butter, cheese and other dairy products as well as animal fat in meat) produces high oestrogen (a female sex hormone) levels due to specific bacteria in the intestine. These raised oestrogen levels have a possible bearing on the incidence of breast cancer. Also it is known that women who are overweight are more prone to breast cancer than their slimmer sisters. So here again dietary factors can be implicated—as well as, of course—large breasts being more difficult to examine adequately than smaller breasts.

The role of oestrogen, and other related hormones in breast cancer is an interesting one in which active research is progressing. Basically, some breast cancers are dependent on these kind of hormones for growth, while others are not. If the cancer cells do need these hormones, there are drugs available which can counteract this, and so be an added form of available treatment. The subject is a complex one needing much further work.

A high-fibre diet can also be postulated to be beneficial. The specific bacteria which help to produce higher levels of oestrogen in the gut may be present in smaller amounts in a high-fibre diet. There has been no proven research done to substantiate this theory at present. But a low-fat, high-fibre diet is beneficial for many reasons anyway. The link with breast cancer, however tenuous, may be just one more reason for an alteration in western society's dietary habits.

These then are some of the factors which are possibly involved in the development of breast cancer in women. It would seem at first sight that there is little that any one specific woman can do in practical terms. But a change to a healthier diet, deliberately choosing to breastfeed her babies—on a demand basis—and choosing to have her family earlier rather than later are perhaps factors worth considering when reviewing lifestyle. Add to this the importance of detecting early disease by the variety of methods discussed, and women will be doing as much as they can to reduce the incidence of this unpleasant disease.

## Signs and symptoms of breast cancer

1 In over 90 per cent of breast cancers a lump has been the first thing noticed. This is usually painless and is not tender when touched. It has a specific 'feel'—usually hard with irregular edges—with which skilled fingers used to palpating breast lumps will be familiar. The upper, outer quarter of either breast is the commonest position for a breast cancer. (But this does not mean that the rest of the breast should receive scant attention during your periodic self-examination.)

2 The next most common symptom, after the finding of a lump, is a discharge from the nipple. This may be

bloodstained, but can also consist of a clear, yellowish fluid.

3 Other symptoms are:

- Pulling to one side of the nipple.
- Wrinkling or ulceration of the skin over an underlying lump.
- Lumps under the arm.
- Swellings or pain in other parts of the body (due to spread of the disease).

These all point to a more advanced stage of the disease. Regular, routine examinations of the breasts will ensure that these later stages are rarely seen.

Any of these signs and symptoms should send you to your doctor. He will examine you and decide whether or not further advice from a specialist is necessary. But never let fear or worry distract you from seeking medical advice. If your particular lump is not cancerous you are worrying unnecessarily and treatment will help the condition. If your lump *is* cancerous, you are giving yourself, and the doctors caring for you, the very best possible chance of cure by attending for treatment early.

## Steps taken to confirm diagnosis

*Examination*
Doctor and specialist will examine your breast thoroughly. Experienced fingers can tell, with a fair degree of accuracy, whether the lump is cancerous or not. Special attention will be paid to the *lymph nodes* in the armpit. Spread to these structures will influence the treatment of the disease. (Various 'stages' of development of the tumour are decided upon, as this will also determine the best form of treatment.)

*Biopsy*
This can take two forms. The first is an *aspiration biopsy*, in which fluid from a cystic swelling is taken for examination

under the microscope. This is done under a local anaesthetic. The arrangement and type of cells seen will assist the surgeon in deciding what form of treatment will need to be envisaged. The drawback to this form of biopsy is that the needle may miss a part of the swelling that contains cancerous cells and so a false picture is given. In view of this, it is necessary for a further biopsy of either the whole lump or a part of it to be taken. Sections of this are looked at under the microscope, and in this way the diagnosis can be firmly made. This is often done in the laboratory quickly while the woman is still under the anaesthetic. Biopsy scars are small and heal quickly with a minimum of disfigurement. They are done in a radial fashion into the breast tissue to avoid any pulling and stretching.

At first sight, an aspiration biopsy would seem to be a waste of time in that a negative result is not necessarily accepted. But this test must firstly be taken in conjunction with all other examinations—namely the initial clinical examination by a skilled doctor. Second, if the test should prove positive, this gives much help to the surgeon planning his regime of treatment. Also, from the woman's point of view, time can be taken to discuss with her doctor the implications of all forms of treatment, and also allow her to come to terms with the possible loss of her breast, rather than waking up after a general anaesthetic to find it removed.

*Mammography and ultrasound*
These may also be used in conjunction with other tests to give further help with planned treatment (see pages 76–9).

## Treatment for breast cancer

There are several forms of treatment for this condition. Surgeons vary in the form of treatment they advise—so women living in one country, or even different parts of the same country, may well be advised on differing forms of treatment. No one treatment, or combinations of treatment, has been proved to give better results than another. Each woman must rely on, and trust in, the doctors who are caring for her. They will have full knowledge of the stage which her disease has reached as well as full understanding of all the treatments available. The 'staging' of the disease (that is, the size and position of the growth and whether or not it has spread locally or to other organs of the body) is an important aspect to be considered when planning a treatment regime. A number of disciplines must work together to ensure that all available facilities, drugs and other forms of treatment can be planned to give the best possible result in each individual woman. So, if this should happen to you, do not be annoyed or distressed if you are sent to see a number of specialists.

The people it is possible that you may see are:

1 Your *own doctor*, who will refer you to a *surgeon*. This surgeon will be the one in your particular district who has chosen to specialize in this type of work—that is, breast cancer—in addition to his general surgical skills. So be reassured that he is fully conversant with all available techniques and additional forms of treatment. This surgeon will probably be the person who oversees whatever form of treatment may be decided upon.

2 A *radiologist*, a doctor who has specialized in irradiation as a form of treatment for many differing forms of cancer. His skills are frequently used in close conjunction with those of the surgeon.

3 A *physician* who has specialized in all forms of treatment —other than surgery—for cancer of all kinds. He will advise on, and prescribe, any drugs which may be thought necessary to control the disease.

4 Any number of dedicated *nurses, radiotherapists* and *physiotherapists* who will be assisting in delivering the appropriate form of treatment to you. Add to this, *community nurses* and members of such organizations as the Mastectomy Association (see page 95) and you will see that there are very many people who are concerned, with you, in your fight against breast cancer.

A look at the role and activity of each of these specialists will give an idea of the scope of treatment available for breast cancer.

### Your own doctor

He, or she, will be the person to whom you will initially go as soon as you discover a lump in your breast. And do remember that you are the most likely person to discover this. An annual check will only tell you that your breast is clear of disease at that particular moment in time. It may be the very next week or month that a lump may become obvious. So by the time your next annual check comes round—if you are lucky enough to have this service available where you live—*your* lump will be that much bigger.

After referring you to a surgeon, your own doctor will be kept informed of the course of treatment you are being advised to follow. And it is to him that you must turn if you are concerned about any side-effects of treatment or worries that you may have between visits to the specialists concerned in your care. So, your own family practitioner could be described as your 'home base' throughout treatment —as indeed he is with all other aspects of your health.

### The surgeon

The surgeon will first of all carefully examine your breasts. He will also examine the rest of your body to exclude spread of the disease to other organs. With his long experience and skilled fingers he will then be able to begin to formulate a plan of campaign, should he suspect that your particular lump is cancerous. He may decide that biopsy—of whatever type—will be most profitable, and/or mammography and ultrasound to give him further clues as to the form and extent of the disease.

In the vast majority of cases, surgery of one form or another is necessary for breast cancer. There are various forms of this procedure and each surgeon will have as his favourite the form which, in his experience, has proved to be the most valuable. The method used will, of course, be dependent on the size and staging of the cancer. Types of surgery are the following:

1 A *lumpectomy* which, as the name implies, is the removal of the lump only. This is carried out under a general anaesthetic, and will leave the breast intact, with only a small scar, which quickly fades in most cases.
2 A *segmental mastectomy*. This is the removal of a segment, or wedge, of breast tissue surrounding the lump. This is infrequently performed, as results have not been found to be as good as other forms of surgery. But there are women around alive and well many years after this form of treatment.
3 A *simple mastectomy*. This is where the whole of the breast is removed. Usually, the lymph nodes in the armpit are also removed at the same time; but the underlying chest muscles are left intact, so that there is no deforming 'hollowness' of the chest after surgery. This is probably the most usual form of surgical procedure.
4 A *radical mastectomy*. This is the operation in which, as well as removal of the breast, there is extensive removal of the chest wall muscles and lymph nodes in a wide surrounding area. This can lead to problems with swelling of the arm due to poor lymph drainage afterwards, as well as being a disfiguring operation. But by this procedure, as much as possible of potentially cancerous tissue—due to spread—is removed.
5 Of increasing popularity is the *subcutaneous mastectomy*. Here the lump and surrounding breast tissue are dissected out, leaving the overlying skin. An 'implant' is then inserted—either during the course of the initial operation or at a later date. By this means the shape of the breast is maintained and deformity is nil or minimal.

There is no 'right' or 'wrong' surgical procedure. Much will depend on the size and staging of the tumour as well as the surgeon's own preference. All women should be fully conversant with what the surgeon proposes to do with their particular cancer. Time must be given for full explanation and discussion.

*The radiologist*
The *radiologist* is the doctor who will be involved in any radiation treatment that is thought to be necessary following surgery to the breast. Close co-operation with the surgeon is necessary in planning the treatment. A number of short visits to a regional centre, two or three times a week, usually over a number of weeks, is the usual form of practice.

Radiation therapy is a painless treatment, although there may be a few side-effects.

1  The skin over the area irradiated can become reddened and slightly itchy, rather like sunburn. Women are advised to avoid washing the part of the body exposed to the irradiation during the course of treatment, as this can exacerbate the potential skin problems. Trauma— scratching, rubbing, bumping—of this part of the body should be avoided as far as possible during treatment.
2  Tiny threads of raised blood vessels can also sometimes arise over the irradiated area. These will disappear within a few weeks once treatment has stopped.
3  Occasionally, some women suffer from a cough and some shortness of breath can result temporarily. This is due to the effects of the radiation on the underlying lung, but it will soon clear at the conclusion of treatment.

*The physician*
A physician who specializes in the treatment of cancer in all its various aspects may be involved in the care of a woman with cancer of her breast. This form of treatment is based on the ability of powerful drugs to kill all cancer cells in the body. This is a splendid idea, but unfortunately many of these drugs also affect normal cells and give rise to many unpleasant side-effects, such as nausea and loss of hair. They are infrequently used in the treatment of cancer of the breast for this reason. Usually only advanced cases of

the disease are thought suitable for this form of chemo-therapy.

Over the last two decades there has been increasing interest in the use of other naturally occurring substances in the body called endocrines. Certain breast tumours have been shown to be responsive to endocrine therapy—some tumour cells will 'bond' to certain drugs which then inhibit further growth of the tumour. To determine if the specific cancer is sensitive to this form of treatment, special tests will need to be done on a sample of the growth. Research is still being actively pursued into this exciting form of treatment for some breast cancers.

*Other professionals*

There are many other professionals involved in the care of the woman having treatment for her breast cancer.

*Nurses* and *radiotherapists*, with their cheerful attitudes and skilled attention, can do so much towards making a worrying time of life more acceptable. And who can measure the effects of an optimistic outlook on the eventual outcome of any disease? The right attitudes and positive thinking can so much be influenced by the quality of care given.

*Physiotherapists* can have an important part to play for women who have had extensive surgery to their breast. If the surgery has involved removal of some of the muscles of the chest, movement of the arm on that side of the body can be difficult and painful initially. But early activity and mobilization of this arm is an important part of getting back to normal. Certain specific exercises—some of which are easier to perform with specialized equipment—with which physiotherapists are familiar can be of great value in this aim.

When you return home from hospital, your *community nurse* (attached to your doctor's practice) may need to visit you to dress the wound, and maybe to remove stitches if this has not already been done in hospital.

## The Mastectomy Association

The Mastectomy Association of Great Britain is a voluntary non-medical organization helping women who have had a mastectomy come to terms with the loss of a breast. They also provide information and practical help. Examples of this latter aspect of their work is advice that can be given about false breasts (prostheses) and suitable specialized clothing, such as bras and swimwear. There is a nationwide network of women who have had a recent mastectomy who are willing and able to talk to other women about to undergo the operation or who have recently returned home from hospital. They work in close liaison with the hospital services and many nurses and social workers are involved. The address of the Mastectomy Association is:

26 Harrison Street (off Grays Inn Road)
Kings Cross, London WC1H 8JG.
Telephone (01) 837 0908.

The Mastectomy Association does not provide breast prostheses, but can give advice to women on this subject. Following a mastectomy, every woman is entitled to be fitted with a free prosthesis on the National Health Service. Occasionally it has proved difficult for women to obtain and be fitted with a suitable prosthesis. Here the Mastectomy Association can advise on the types available (there are currently fourteen different types, so finding one to suit each individual woman should be possible). Any difficulties obtaining a suitable breast replacement should be referred back to the consultant who performed the mastectomy.

## Coming to terms with breast cancer

Breast cancer is an unpleasant disease. In addition to the purely physical aspects of the condition go the undoubtedly psychological upsets that most women have to face particularly when a mastectomy is advised. In spite of a seeming increase in the number of women suffering from a breast cancer (possibly because women feel more able to discuss their conditions these days) there has been no overall increase in the incidence of breast cancer in recent years. As with cancers of other types, breast cancer becomes more common with increasing age. The fact must be faced that thousands of women will die from breast cancer every year. But it cannot be too highly stressed—and acted upon—that early treatment gives the best chance of cure. Today's treatments have progressed—and are progressing—from those of even a decade ago. So treatment need not be dreaded. Also the after-effects of treatment are improving yearly, so that the quality of life following treatment for breast cancer is also vastly improved.

Finally, much money is still being given to research into breast cancer. Hopefully one day a way of preventing this feminine scourge will be found.

# APPENDIX

# Conditions of the Male Breast

No book on the breast is complete without a brief mention of conditions which can affect the masculine breast. Fortunately these conditions are rare when compared with the multitude of conditions that can affect the female breast.

The breast in men is something of an evolutionary puzzle. It would seem to fulfil no obvious useful function—so why should men have minimal breasts and nipples?

Male breasts consist of fatty tissue, blood vessels, and ducts (but not glandular milk-producing cells as in the female breast) beneath the typical nipple and—smaller—areola area. As men's bodies do not undergo cyclical monthly changes as do those of women, there are no conditions such as breast tenderness and enlargement which are the common feminine experience.

Abnormalities of breast development can occur in the male breast as in the female. For example, a number of 'breasts' (often looking rather like 'moles') can be present along the milk ridges of baby boys. These will cause no problem as they may in girls, where at puberty further development may take place.

Baby boys can suffer as often with breast enlargement and secretion of milk as do baby girls. This 'witch's milk' is due to the high level of female hormones passed on from their mothers. The enlargement—or *gynaemastia*—will disappear quite spontaneously, although this may take several weeks to finally resolve. Very rarely will infection intervene, needing antibiotic treatment. Similarly, during the years of puberty, enlargement of the male breast can occur. This is again due to hormonal influences, and will eventually subside once the boy's hormonal levels have stabilized. He will, however, need much support from family and friends through these months, as he may well experience much teasing, and subsequent psychological upset, from his contemporaries. The true cause for his enlarged breasts must be freely explained to him or he may have worries, rarely voiced, about his masculinity.

There are other, rare diseases which can cause this type of breast enlargement in men. But with these there will be other more obvious symptoms of the main disease.

Cancer of the breast can occur in men—albeit rarely. As there is comparatively little fatty tissue, any small swelling is noticeable and so diagnosis, followed by treatment, is usually earlier than in many women. Discharge from the nipple is often an early symptom in cancer of the male breast. Treatment is along similar lines as for female breast cancer, and early treatment, as with all cancers, holds the best chance of cure.

The male breast is usually disease free. However, the occasional problems can arise, some needing treatment, but other troubles resolve themselves spontaneously.

# Index